Hemodynamic Monitoring

made Incredibly Visual!™

Third Edition

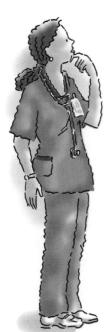

Rose Knapp, DNP, RN, APRN-BC
Assistant Graduate Faculty
APN Program Coordinator
Monmouth University
Marjorie K Unterberg School of Nursing and Health Studies
West Long Branch, NJ

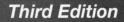
®. Wolters Kluwer

Philadelphia • Baltimore • New York • London
Buenos Aires • Hong Kong • Sydney • Tokyo

Executive Editor: Shannon W. Magee
Product Development Editor: Maria M. McAvey
Senior Marketing Manager: Mark Wiragh
Production Project Manager: Marian Bellus
Design Coordinator: Elaine Kasmer
Manufacturing Coordinator: Kathleen Brown
Prepress Vendor: S4Carlisle Publishing Services

Library of Congress Cataloging-in-Publication Data
Hemodynamic monitoring made incredibly visual / Rose Knapp. — Third edition.
     pages cm
  Includes bibliographical references and index.
  ISBN 978-1-4963-0699-9 (alk. paper)
  1. Hemodynamic monitoring—Atlases.   2. Cardiovascular system—Diseases—Diagnosis—Atlases.
3. Patient monitoring—Atlases.   4. Nursing—Atlases.   I. Knapp, Rose.
  RC670.5.H45H46 2016
  616.1'0754—dc23

                                                                                        2015020117

Dedication

To all critical care nurses who work tirelessly to care of our hemodynamically challenged patient population.

To my family John, Kristina, and Stephanie for all of their support over the years.

Contributors

Susan Barnason, PhD, RN, APRN-CNS, CEN, CCRN, FAEN, FAHA, FAAN
Professor of Nursing
University of Nebraska Medical Center
College of Nursing
Lincoln, NE

Natalie Burkhalter, RN, MSM, CS, FNP, ACNP
Family Nurse Practitioner
Mercy Ministries of Laredo
Laredo, TX

Kathleen M. Hill, MSN, RN, CCNS
Clinical Nurse Specialist, Surgical
  Intensive Care Unit
Cleveland Clinic
Cleveland, OH

Julene B. (Julie) Kruithof, MSN, RN, CCRN
Adult Critical Care Educator
Spectrum Health
Grand Rapids, MI

Margaret McAtee, RN, ACNP-BC, CCRN
Cardiovascular Nurse Practitioner
Baylor All Saints Medical Center
Fort Worth, TX

Nancy M. Richards, RN, MSN, CCRN, CCNS
Cardiovascular Surgery Clinical Nurse
  Specialist and Ventricular Assist Device
  (VAD) Coordinator
Saint Luke's Hospital
Kansas City, MO

Maria E. Rodriguez, DNP, ACNS-BC
Nursing Educator
Walden University
Department of Nursing
Minneapolis, MN

Michelle D. Staggs, APN, ACNP-BC, CCRN, CEN, TNS
Acute Care Nurse Practitioner
Southwest Pulmonary Associates
Little Rock, AR

Loisann Stapleton, RN, MSN, CCRN, APN-C
Acute Care Nurse Practitioner
Atlantic Cardiology, L.L.C.
Neptune, NJ

Patricia Walters, RN, MSN, APN, CCRN
Nurse Practitioner—Cardiothoracic
  Surgery
Hackensack University Medical Center
Hackensack, NJ

Previous Edition Contributors

Susan Barnason, PhD, RN, APRN-CNS, CEN, CCRN, FAEN, FAHA, FAAN

Natalie Burkhalter, RN, MSM, CS, FNP, ACNP

Kathleen M. Hill, MSN, RN, CCNS

Julene B. (Julie) Kruithof, MSN, RN, CCRN

Margaret McAtee, RN, ACNP-BC, CCRN

Nancy M. Richards, RN, MSN, CCRN, CCNS

Maria E. Rodriguez, DNP, ACNS-BC

Michelle D. Staggs, APN, ACNP-BC, CCRN, CEN, TNS

Patricia Walters, RN, MSN, APN, CCRN

Susan L. Woods, PhD, RN, FAHA, FAAN

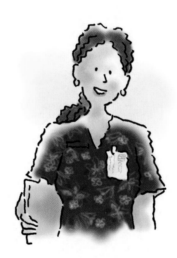

Acknowledgments

To my colleagues who contributed their expertise in cardiovascular nursing to this text:

Susan Barnason, Natalie Burkhalter, Kathleen M. Hill, Julene B. (Julie) Kruithof, Margaret McAtee, Nancy M. Richards, Maria E. Rodriguez, Michelle D. Staggs, Loisann Stapleton, and Patricia Walters

Contents

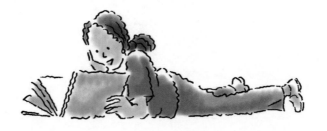

Chapter 1

Cardiopulmonary anatomy and physiology

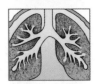

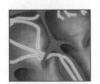

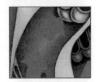

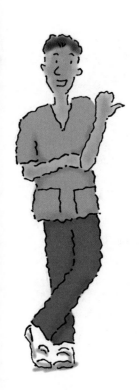

Understanding the pulmonary system

The pulmonary system delivers oxygen to the bloodstream and removes excess carbon dioxide from the body. The alveoli are the gas-exchange units of the lungs. The lungs in a typical adult contain about 300 million alveoli.

A closer look at alveoli

Gas exchange occurs rapidly in the tiny, thin-membraned alveoli. Inside these air sacs, oxygen from inhaled air diffuses into the blood as carbon dioxide diffuses from the blood into the air and is exhaled.

Alveoli consist of type I and type II epithelial cells:
• Type I cells form the alveolar walls, through which gas exchange occurs.
• Type II cells produce surfactant, a lipid-type substance that coats the alveoli. During inspiration, the alveolar surfactant allows the alveoli to expand uniformly. During expiration, the surfactant prevents alveolar collapse.

This illustration shows a cross-section view of an alveolus.

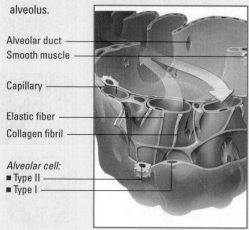

Alveolar duct
Smooth muscle
Capillary
Elastic fiber
Collagen fibril
Alveolar cell:
■ Type II
■ Type I

Structure of intrapulmonary airways

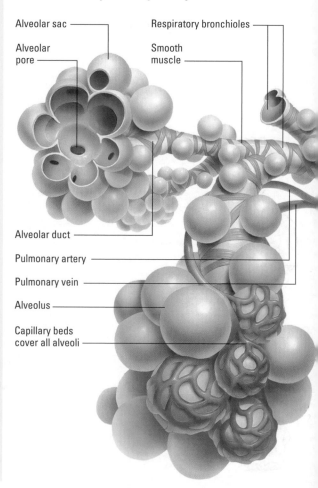

Alveolar sac
Alveolar pore
Respiratory bronchioles
Smooth muscle
Alveolar duct
Pulmonary artery
Pulmonary vein
Alveolus
Capillary beds cover all alveoli

Structures of the pulmonary system

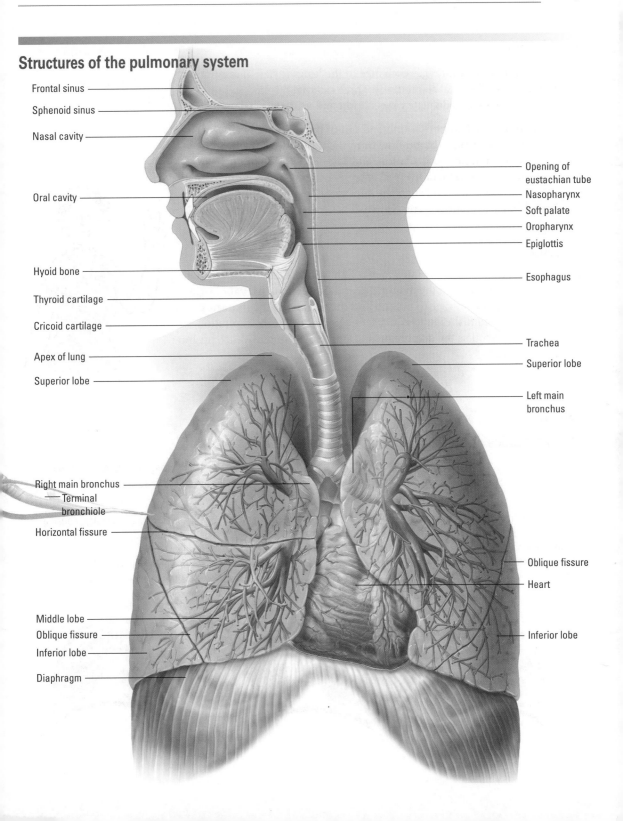

Frontal sinus

Sphenoid sinus

Nasal cavity

Oral cavity

Hyoid bone

Thyroid cartilage

Cricoid cartilage

Apex of lung

Superior lobe

Right main bronchus

Terminal bronchiole

Horizontal fissure

Middle lobe

Oblique fissure

Inferior lobe

Diaphragm

Opening of eustachian tube

Nasopharynx

Soft palate

Oropharynx

Epiglottis

Esophagus

Trachea

Superior lobe

Left main bronchus

Oblique fissure

Heart

Inferior lobe

Respiration

Effective respiration requires gas exchange in the lungs (external respiration) and in the tissues (internal respiration). Three external respiration processes are needed to maintain adequate oxygenation and acid–base balance:

1. **Ventilation** (gas distribution into and out of the pulmonary airways)
2. **Pulmonary perfusion** (blood flow from the right side of the heart, through the pulmonary circulation, and into the left side of the heart)
3. **Diffusion** (gas movement from an area of greater concentration to an area of lesser concentration through a semipermeable membrane) Blood enters the pulmonary cap deoxygenated which has lower partial pressure of O_2 in inhaled alveolar air

> Ventilation, pulmonary perfusion, and diffusion are the three processes for adequate oxygenation and acid–base balance.

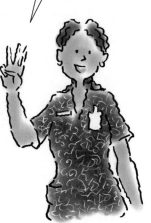

Ventilation

Breathing, or *ventilation*, is the movement of air into and out of the respiratory system. During inspiration, the diaphragm and external intercostal muscles contract, causing the rib cage to expand and the volume of the thoracic cavity to increase. Air then rushes in to equalize the pressure. During expiration, the lungs passively recoil as the diaphragm and intercostal muscles relax, pushing air out of the lungs.

The mechanics of breathing

Mechanical forces, such as movement of the diaphragm and intercostal muscles, drive the breathing process. In these depictions, a plus sign (+) indicates positive pressure and a minus sign (–) indicates negative pressure.

At rest
• Inspiratory muscles relax.
• Atmospheric pressure is maintained in the tracheobronchial tree.
• No air movement occurs.

Inspiration
• Inspiratory muscles contract.
• The diaphragm descends.
• Negative alveolar pressure is maintained.

Expiration
• Inspiratory muscles relax, causing lungs to recoil to their resting size and position.
• The diaphragm ascends.
• Positive alveolar pressure is maintained.

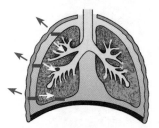
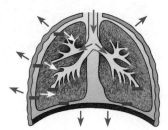
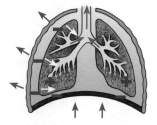

Pulmonary perfusion

Blood flow through the lungs is powered by the right ventricle. The right and left pulmonary arteries carry deoxygenated blood from the right ventricle to the lungs. These arteries divide to form distal branches called *arterioles*, which terminate as a concentrated capillary network in the alveoli and alveolar sac, where gas exchange occurs.

Venules—the end branches of the pulmonary veins—collect oxygenated blood from the capillaries and transport it to larger vessels, which carry it to the pulmonary veins. The pulmonary veins enter the left side of the heart and distribute oxygenated blood throughout the body.

Tracking pulmonary perfusion

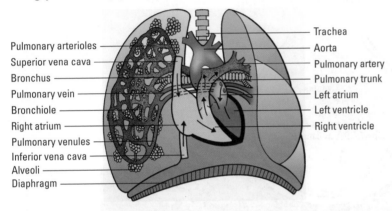

Pulmonary arterioles
Superior vena cava
Bronchus
Pulmonary vein
Bronchiole
Right atrium
Pulmonary venules
Inferior vena cava
Alveoli
Diaphragm

Trachea
Aorta
Pulmonary artery
Pulmonary trunk
Left atrium
Left ventricle
Right ventricle

Understanding PVR

Pulmonary vascular resistance (PVR) refers to the resistance in the pulmonary vascular bed against which the right ventricle must eject blood. PVR is largely determined by the caliber and degree of tone of the pulmonary arteries, capillaries, and veins and is measured with the use of hemodynamic monitoring. Because these vessels are thin-walled and highly elastic, PVR is normally very low. However, PVR may be easily influenced by vasoactive stimuli that dilate or constrict the pulmonary vessels or affect the tone of these vessels.

Factors that increase PVR include:
➢ vasoconstricting drugs
➢ hypoxemia
➢ acidemia
➢ hypercapnia
➢ atelectasis.

Factors that decrease PVR include:
➢ vasodilating drugs
➢ alkalemia
➢ hypocapnia
➢ conditions that result in high cardiac output, such as during strenuous exercise.

Diffusion

Blood in the pulmonary capillaries gains oxygen and loses carbon dioxide through the process of diffusion (gas exchange). In this process, oxygen and carbon dioxide move from an area of greater concentration to an area of lesser concentration through the pulmonary capillary, a semipermeable membrane. This illustration shows how the differences in gas concentration between blood in the pulmonary artery (deoxygenated blood from the right side of the heart) and alveolus make this process possible. Gas concentrations depicted in the pulmonary vein are the end result of gas exchange and represent the blood that is delivered to the left side of the heart and systemic circulation.

Diffusion across the alveolar–capillary membrane

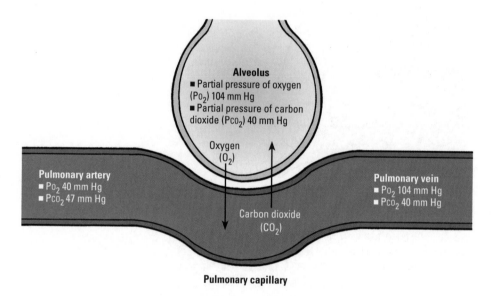

Alveolus
- Partial pressure of oxygen (Po_2) 104 mm Hg
- Partial pressure of carbon dioxide (Pco_2) 40 mm Hg

Oxygen (O_2)

Pulmonary artery
- Po_2 40 mm Hg
- Pco_2 47 mm Hg

Pulmonary vein
- Po_2 104 mm Hg
- Pco_2 40 mm Hg

Carbon dioxide (CO_2)

Pulmonary capillary

Ventilation and perfusion ratio

Areas where perfusion and ventilation are similar have a ventilation–perfusion ($\dot{V}/\dot{Q}$) match. Gas exchange is most efficient in such areas. For example, in normal lung function, the alveoli receive air at a rate of about 4 L/min while the capillaries supply blood to the alveoli at a rate of about 5 L/min, creating a ($\dot{V}/\dot{Q}$) ratio of 4:5, or 0.8 (the normal range for a ($\dot{V}/\dot{Q}$) ratio is from 0.8 to 1.2).

A ($\dot{V}/\dot{Q}$) mismatch, resulting from ventilation–perfusion dysfunction or altered lung mechanics, indicates ineffective gas exchange between the alveoli and pulmonary capillaries, and can affect all body systems by changing the amount of oxygen delivered to living cells.

Understanding ventilation and perfusion

Key

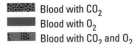

Blood with CO_2
Blood with O_2
Blood with CO_2 and O_2

Causes

Conditions that may produce a V̇/Q̇ mismatch include:

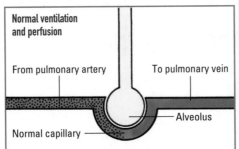

Normal ventilation and perfusion

From pulmonary artery

To pulmonary vein

Alveolus

Normal capillary

When ventilation and perfusion (V̇/Q̇) are matched, unoxygenated blood from the venous system returns to the right side of the heart through the pulmonary artery to the lungs, carrying carbon dioxide (CO_2). The arteries branch into the alveolar capillaries. Gas exchange takes place in the alveolar capillaries.

1 *Shunting* (reduced ventilation to a lung unit) causes unoxygenated blood to move from the right side of the heart to the left side of the heart and into systemic circulation; it may result from physical defects or airway obstruction.

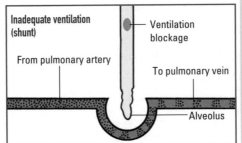

Inadequate ventilation (shunt)

Ventilation blockage

From pulmonary artery

To pulmonary vein

Alveolus

When the V̇/Q̇ ratio is low, pulmonary circulation is adequate, but not enough oxygen (O_2) is available to the alveoli for normal diffusion. A portion of the blood flowing through the pulmonary vessels does not become oxygenated.

2 *Dead-space ventilation* (reduced perfusion to a lung unit) occurs when alveoli do not have adequate blood supply for gas exchange to occur, such as with pulmonary emboli and pulmonary infarction.

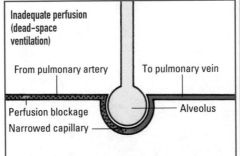

Inadequate perfusion (dead-space ventilation)

From pulmonary artery

To pulmonary vein

Perfusion blockage

Narrowed capillary

Alveolus

When the V̇/Q̇ ratio is high, as shown here, ventilation is normal, but alveolar perfusion is reduced or absent. Note the narrowed capillary, indicating poor perfusion. This commonly results from a perfusion defect, such as pulmonary embolism or a disorder that decreases cardiac output.

3 *A silent unit* (a combination of shunting and dead-space ventilation) occurs when little or no ventilation and perfusion are present, such as in cases of pneumothorax and acute respiratory distress syndrome.

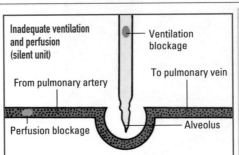

Inadequate ventilation and perfusion (silent unit)

Ventilation blockage

From pulmonary artery

To pulmonary vein

Perfusion blockage

Alveolus

The silent unit indicates an absence of ventilation and perfusion to the lung area. The silent unit may help compensate a V̇/Q̇ imbalance by delivering blood flow to better ventilated lung areas.

Understanding the cardiac system

The cardiac system:

■ carries life-sustaining oxygen and nutrients in the blood to all cells of the body

■ removes metabolic waste products in the blood from the cells.

The heart is a cone-shaped muscle that pumps the body's entire volume of blood to the lungs (right ventricle) and all of the other organs (left ventricle). The major blood vessels of the heart are the left and right coronary arteries, which branch from the base of the aorta.

A closer look at the heart

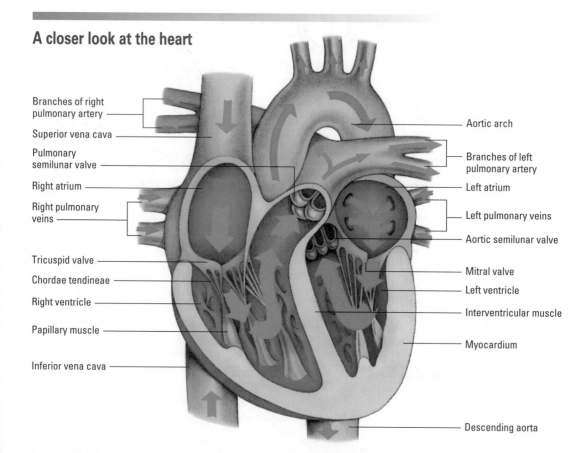

Branches of right pulmonary artery

Superior vena cava

Pulmonary semilunar valve

Right atrium

Right pulmonary veins

Tricuspid valve

Chordae tendineae

Right ventricle

Papillary muscle

Inferior vena cava

Aortic arch

Branches of left pulmonary artery

Left atrium

Left pulmonary veins

Aortic semilunar valve

Mitral valve

Left ventricle

Interventricular muscle

Myocardium

Descending aorta

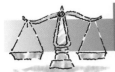

On the level

Normal intracardiac pressures

Structure	Normal pressure
Right atrium	0 to 8 mm Hg
Right ventricle	Systolic: 15 to 25 mm Hg Diastolic: 0 to 8 mm Hg
Pulmonary artery	Systolic: 15 to 25 mm Hg Diastolic: 8 to 15 mm Hg
Left atrium	4 to 12 mm Hg
Left ventricle	Systolic: 110 to 130 mm Hg Diastolic: 4 to 12 mm Hg
Aorta	Systolic: 110 to 130 mm Hg Diastolic: 70 to 80 mm Hg

These two views of the heart might help you put together the pieces of the heart puzzle! They show the great vessels and some major coronary vessels.

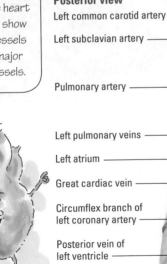

Viewing coronary vessels

Anterior view

Left subclavian artery

Left common carotid artery

Brachiocephalic artery

Aortic arch

Superior vena cava

Pulmonary trunk

Right atrium

Right coronary artery

Great cardiac vein

Circumflex branch of left coronary artery

Small cardiac vein

Anterior interventricular (descending) branch of left main coronary artery

Posterior view

Left common carotid artery

Left subclavian artery

Pulmonary artery

Left pulmonary veins

Left atrium

Great cardiac vein

Circumflex branch of left coronary artery

Posterior vein of left ventricle

Middle cardiac vein

Brachiocephalic artery

Aortic arch

Superior vena cava

Right pulmonary veins

Right atrium

Inferior vena cava

Small cardiac vein

Right coronary artery

Posterior interventricular (descending) branch of right coronary artery

Cardiac conduction

The conduction system of the heart begins with the heart's pacemaker, the sinoatrial (SA) node. When an impulse leaves the SA node, it travels through the atria along Bachmann's bundle and the internodal pathways on its way to the atrioventricular (AV) node and the ventricles. After the impulse passes through the AV node, it travels to the ventricles, first down the bundle of His, then along the bundle branches, and, lastly, down the Purkinje fibers.

Cardiac conduction system

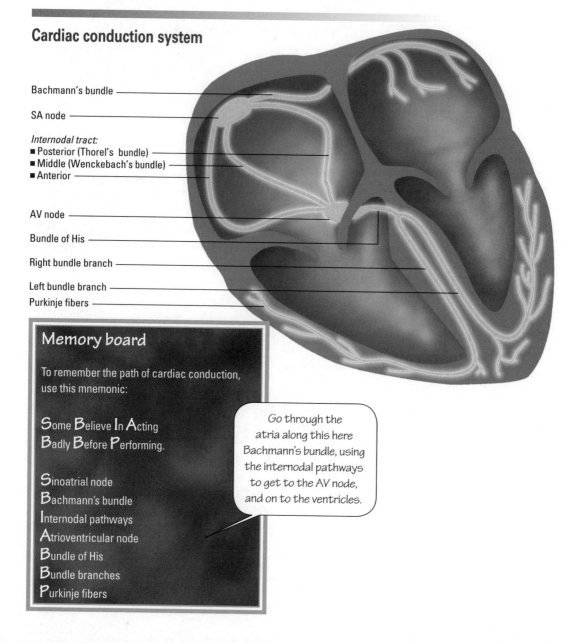

Bachmann's bundle

SA node

Internodal tract:
- Posterior (Thorel's bundle)
- Middle (Wenckebach's bundle)
- Anterior

AV node

Bundle of His

Right bundle branch

Left bundle branch

Purkinje fibers

Memory board

To remember the path of cardiac conduction, use this mnemonic:

Some **B**elieve **I**n **A**cting
Badly **B**efore **P**erforming.

Sinoatrial node
Bachmann's bundle
Internodal pathways
Atrioventricular node
Bundle of His
Bundle branches
Purkinje fibers

Go through the atria along this here Bachmann's bundle, using the internodal pathways to get to the AV node, and on to the ventricles.

Events of the cardiac cycle

1 Isovolumetric ventricular contraction
In response to ventricular depolarization, tension in the ventricles increases. This rise in pressure within the ventricles leads to closure of the mitral and tricuspid valves. The pulmonic and aortic valves stay closed during the entire phase.

2 Ventricular ejection
When ventricular pressure exceeds aortic and pulmonary arterial pressure, the aortic and pulmonic valves open and the ventricles eject blood.

5 Atrial systole
Known as the *atrial kick,* atrial systole (coinciding with late ventricular diastole) supplies the ventricles with the remaining 30% of the blood for each heartbeat.

4 Ventricular filling
Atrial pressure exceeds ventricular pressure, which causes the mitral and tricuspid valves to open. Blood then flows passively into the ventricles. About 70% of ventricular filling takes place during this phase.

3 Isovolumetric relaxation
When ventricular pressure falls below the pressure in the aorta and pulmonary artery, the aortic and pulmonic valves close. All valves are closed during this phase. Atrial diastole occurs as blood fills the atria.

Cardiovascular circuit

The cardiovascular circuit is a continuous, closed, fluid-filled elastic system of arteries, capillaries, and veins. The heart acts as a pump for this system.

Blood circulation

Blood enters the right atrium from the vena cava and flows into the right ventricle. Heart muscles contract to send blood through the pulmonary trunk to the lungs for oxygenation. Blood returns to the left atrium through the pulmonary veins and flows into the left ventricle. Heart muscles contract again to drive blood through the aorta into the arterial system of the body. As arteries become increasingly smaller, blood reaches capillary beds where oxygen is released to the cells of organs and tissues. Veins then carry oxygen-poor blood back to the vena cava.

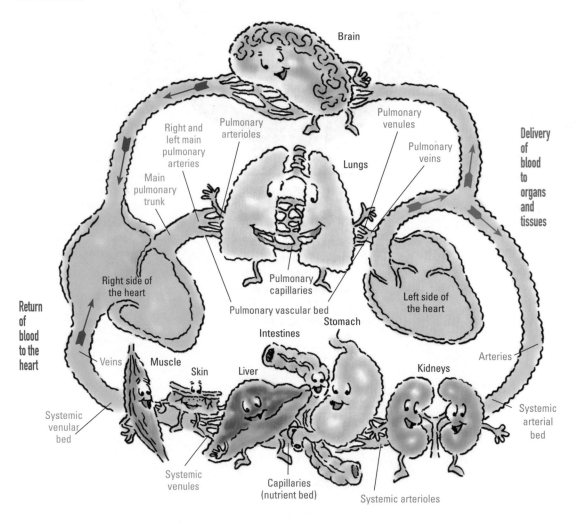

Systemic vascular resistance

Systemic vascular resistance (SVR) represents the resistance against which the left ventricle must pump to move blood throughout systemic circulation. SVR can be affected by:

- tone and diameter of the blood vessels
- viscosity of the blood
- resistance from the inner lining of the blood vessels.

SVR usually has an inverse relationship to cardiac output; that is, when SVR decreases, cardiac output increases, and when cardiac output decreases, SVR will increase.

Although newer electronic monitors can automatically calculate SVR from hemodynamic measurements, the following formula can be used to calculate it by hand:

$$SVR = \frac{\text{mean arterial pressure} - \text{central venous pressure}}{\text{cardiac output}} \times 80$$

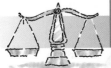

On the level

Measurements of SVR

Normal measurements of SVR range from 770 to 1,500 dynes/sec/cm^{-5}.

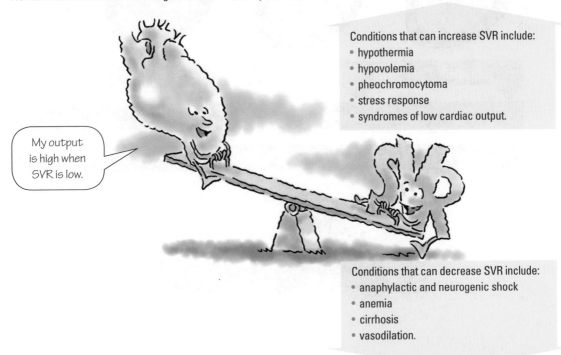

Conditions that can increase SVR include:
- hypothermia
- hypovolemia
- pheochromocytoma
- stress response
- syndromes of low cardiac output.

My output is high when SVR is low.

Conditions that can decrease SVR include:
- anaphylactic and neurogenic shock
- anemia
- cirrhosis
- vasodilation.

Cardiac output

Cardiac output is the amount of blood the heart pumps in 1 minute. It is
equal to the heart rate multiplied by the stroke volume (the amount of blood
ejected with each heartbeat).

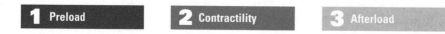

Cardiac output = heart rate × stroke volume

Stroke volume depends on three major factors:

1 Preload   **2** Contractility   **3** Afterload

Influences on stroke volume and cardiac output

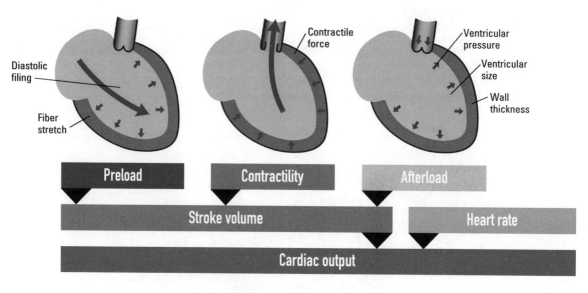

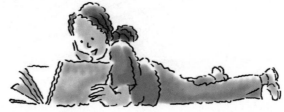

Understanding preload, contractility, and afterload

If you think of the heart as a balloon, it will help you understand preload, contractility, and afterload.

Preload

Preload is the stretching of muscle fibers in the ventricle. This stretching results from blood volume in the ventricles at end-diastole. According to Starling's law, the more the heart muscles stretch during diastole, the more forcefully they contract during systole. Think of preload as the balloon stretching as air is blown into it. The more air, the greater the stretch.

Contractility

Contractility refers to the inherent ability of the myocardium to contract normally. Contractility is influenced by preload. The greater the stretch the more forceful the contraction—or, the more air in the balloon, the greater the stretch, and the farther the balloon will fly when air is allowed to expel.

Afterload

Afterload refers to the pressure that the ventricular muscles must generate to overcome the higher pressure in the aorta to get the blood out of the heart. Resistance is the knot on the end of the balloon, which the balloon has to work against to get the air out.

This chart might show the effects of preload and afterload, but I think you can tell by looking at me what happens when my work increases...

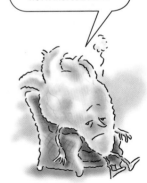

Effects of preload and afterload on the heart

Factor	Possible cause	Effects on heart
Increased preload	• Increased fluid volume • Vasoconstriction	• Increases stroke volume • Increases ventricular work • Increases myocardial oxygen requirements
Decreased preload	• Hypovolemia • Vasodilation	• Decreases stroke volume • Decreases ventricular work • Decreases myocardial oxygen requirements
Increased afterload	• Hypovolemia • Vasoconstriction	• Decreases stroke volume • Increases ventricular work • Increases myocardial oxygen requirements
Decreased afterload	• Vasodilation	• Increases stroke volume • Decreases ventricular work • Decreases myocardial oxygen requirements

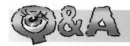

Color my world

Trace the path of blood flow through the heart. Color sections blue where deoxygenated blood flows and red where oxygenated blood flows.

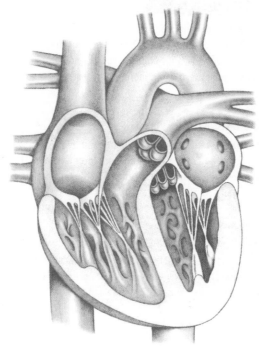

Matchmaker

Match each term to the definitions provided.

1. cardiac output _____   A. The pressure that the ventricular muscles must generate to overcome the higher pressure in the aorta

2. stroke volume _____   B. The stretching of muscle fibers in the ventricle

3. preload _____   C. The amount of blood the heart pumps in 1 minute

4. afterload _____   D. The amount of blood ejected with each heartbeat

5. contractility _____   E. The inherent ability of the myocardium to contract normally

Matchmaker: 1. C, 2. D, 3. B, 4. A, 5. E.

Answers: Color my world: See illustration on page 8 for correct path of flow and correct colors.

Suggested References

Alspach, J.G. (Ed.). *Core Curriculum for Critical Care Nursing*, 6th ed. Philadelphia: W.B. Saunders Co., 2006.

Carlson, K.K. (Ed.). *AACN Advanced Critical Care Nursing*. Philadelphia: Elsevier, 2009.

Chulay, M., and Burns, S.M. *AACN Essentials of Critical Care Nursing*, 3rd ed. New York: McGraw-Hill, 2014.

Diepenbrock, N. *Quick Reference to Critical Care*, 4th ed. Philadelphia: Lippincott Williams & Wilkins, 2012.

McCance, K, and Heuther, S. *Pathoyhysiology: The Biologic Basis for Disease in Adults and Children*, 7th ed. Philadelphia: Elsevier, 2013.

McLaughlin, M.A. (Ed.). *Cardiovascular Care Made Incredibly Easy*, 3rd ed. Philadelphia: Lippincott Williams & Wilkins, 2009.

Stedman's Medical Dictionary for the Health Professions and Nursing, 7th ed. Philadelphia: Wolters Kluwer, 2011.

Morris, T.A., and Fedullo, P.F. Pulmonary thromboembolism. In: Mason, R.J. et al., (Eds.). *Textbook of Respiratory Medicine*, 5th ed. Philadelphia: Saunders Elsevier, 2010:chap 51.

Mosby's Medical Dictionary, 8th ed. Philadelphia: Elsevier, 2009.

Chapter 2

Understanding a pressure monitoring system

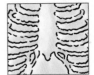

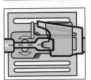

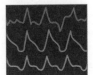

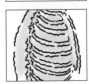

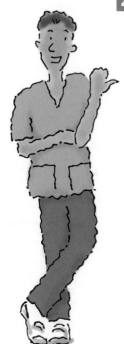

Components of a pressure monitoring system

Hemodynamic monitoring is used to:
- diagnose, manage, and treat cardiopulmonary insufficiency
- manage and treat shock
- assess pulmonary vascular function
- assess cardiac function

It's performed by using a pressure monitoring system to measure cardiovascular pressures. Let's take a closer look at this system.

Multiple-pressure transducer systems

Multiple-pressure transducer systems can monitor two or more types of pressure, such as pulmonary artery pressure and central venous pressure. Two methods may be used to set up this type of system:

1. Add a second setup (with a separate bag of flush solution, pressure transducer, and cable) to the single-pressure system. Label the lines.
2. Use a Y-type tubing setup with two attached pressure transducers, requiring only one bag of flush solution but two pressure cables.

Pressure transducer

The transducer senses pressure changes that are transmitted from the intravascular space or cardiac chamber to the fluid in the nonpliable pressure tubing through the catheter in the patient, and from the nonpliable pressure tubing to the transducer. These pressure changes are transmitted to the monitor via electrical impulses sent through the transducer cable.

← To catheter

Flush device

The flush device is used to manually flush the system.

A closer look at a pressure monitoring system

IV fluid

A continuous infusion of flush solution (usually normal saline or heparinized normal saline) is placed in a pressure bag that's inflated to 300 mm Hg, maintains a constant pressure through the transducer and flush device, and is kept at a low continuous flow of approximately 3 mL/hr to maintain patency, prevent the backflow of blood, and allow for accurate pressure transmissions.

Pressure monitor

The monitor converts the transducer's electrical signals into a pressure tracing (waveform) and digital value that's displayed on the screen.

This system measures cardiac function and helps determine the effectiveness of therapy.

Three-way stopcock

The three-way stopcock is a device that controls the flow of IV solution through the system.

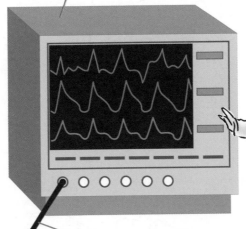

Transducer cable

The transducer cable connects the pressure transducer to the monitor.

Pressure tube

The pressure tubing serves as a connecting tube from the catheter in the patient to the flush device and transducer system. This tubing should be rigid and nonpliable to transmit the most accurate pressure measurements.

Leveling the transducer

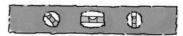

> Nurses use a lot of tools—even a carpenter's level comes in handy for hemodynamic monitoring!

To ensure accurate hemodynamic measurements, the patient and the transducer must be positioned on the same level before the system is zeroed. Leveling involves positioning the air-reference stopcock or the air–fluid interface of the transducer on the same level as the phlebostatic axis. Alternatively, the air-reference stopcock or the air–fluid interface may be leveled to the same position as the catheter tip.

Understanding leveling

1 **Determine the phlebostatic axis**
The phlebostatic axis (level of patient's atria) is the zero-referencing point for the pressure monitoring system. The patient should be lying flat in bed, and the axis is established midway between the posterior chest and the sternum at the fourth intercostal space.

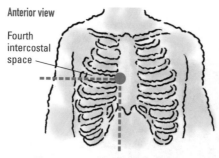

Anterior view

Fourth intercostal space

Lateral view

Outermost point of posterior chest

Outermost point of sternum

2 **Level the system**
Using a carpenter's level, place the air-reference stopcock or the air–fluid interface of the transducer on the same horizontal level with the phlebostatic axis.

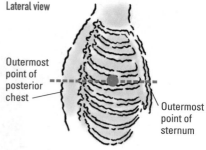

Air-fluid interface

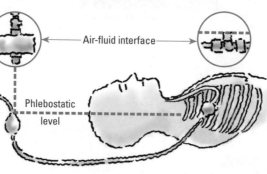

Phlebostatic level

3 **Readjust as necessary**
If the head of the patient's bed is changed (raised or lowered), remember that the reference level will also change. Relevel and zero the system to allow for accurate measurements.

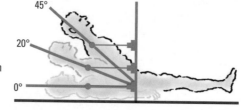

45°

20°

0°

Effects of position changes on hemodynamic measurements

Catheter tip and transducer dome at same vertical level

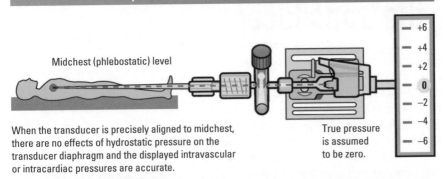

Midchest (phlebostatic) level

When the transducer is precisely aligned to midchest, there are no effects of hydrostatic pressure on the transducer diaphragm and the displayed intravascular or intracardiac pressures are accurate.

True pressure is assumed to be zero.

Air–fluid interface 3" below catheter tip

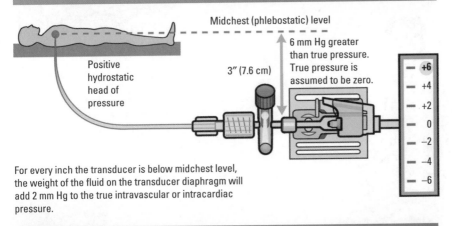

Midchest (phlebostatic) level

Positive hydrostatic head of pressure

3" (7.6 cm)

6 mm Hg greater than true pressure. True pressure is assumed to be zero.

For every inch the transducer is below midchest level, the weight of the fluid on the transducer diaphragm will add 2 mm Hg to the true intravascular or intracardiac pressure.

Air–fluid interface 3" above catheter tip

For every inch the transducer is above midchest level, the displayed intravascular or intracardiac pressure will be about 2 mm Hg less than actual pressures.

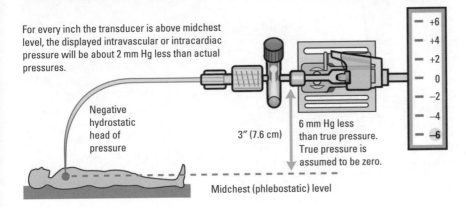

Negative hydrostatic head of pressure

3" (7.6 cm)

6 mm Hg less than true pressure. True pressure is assumed to be zero.

Midchest (phlebostatic) level

Zeroing the transducer

After the pressure monitoring system is leveled, it's time to zero the transducer. Zeroing adjusts the transducer so that it reads zero pressure when it's open to the atmosphere. Zeroing is important because physiologic pressures, such as arterial blood pressure, are relative to the atmospheric pressure. By zeroing the transducer, effects from atmospheric pressure are eliminated and the monitoring system begins pressure measurement at a neutral pressure point of 0 mm Hg. Establishing this neutral point ensures that pressure measurements reflect only the pressure values in the vessel or heart chamber being monitored.

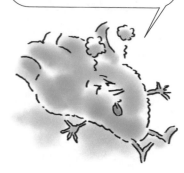

Zeroing the transducer ensures that pressure measurements reflect only the pressure values in my chamber.

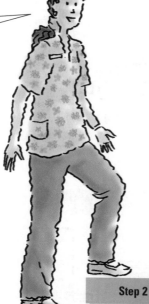

Remember these key steps when zeroing your patient's pressure monitoring system.

Step 1

Level the transducer.

Step 2

Turn the stopcock next to the transducer off to the patient and open to air.

Step 3

Remove the cap to the stopcock port and place it inside an opened sterile gauze package to prevent contamination.

Step 4

Zero the transducer by activating the zero function key on the monitor.

Step 5

When the monitor indicates the system is properly zeroed, replace the stopcock port cap and turn the stopcock so that it's closed to air and open to the patient. Now the monitoring can begin!

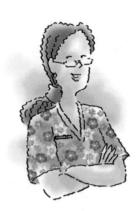

Square wave testing

The square wave test is a simple process performed to evaluate the dynamic response of the pressure monitoring system. If the waveform obtained when performing this test is optimal, you can be assured that the pressure monitoring system is providing accurate pressures and waveforms from the patient.

Performing and interpreting the square wave test

The square wave test is performed by activating the fast-flush device for 1 to 2 seconds and immediately evaluating the configuration on the monitor. The patient's pressure waveform displayed on the monitor will be replaced with a square wave.

Optimally damped system	Overdamped system	Underdamped system

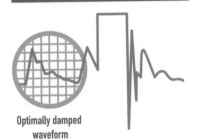

Optimally damped
waveform

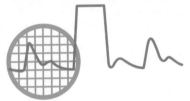

Overdamped
waveform

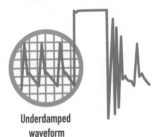

Underdamped
waveform

Characteristics
- Straight vertical upstroke from the baseline
- Straight horizontal component
- Straight vertical downstroke back to baseline with one or two rapid oscillations (most important component)

Interventions
- None required.

Characteristics
- Slurred upstroke and downstroke of the square wave
- No oscillations above or below the baseline

Interventions
- Examine the system from the catheter to the transducer, checking for and eliminating blood clots, blood left in the catheter or tubing following sampling, or air bubbles at any point.
- Be sure to use nonpliable (stiff), pressurized tubing that's less than 4' (1.2 m) long.
- Make sure that all components of the system are connected securely; unravel any kinks in the tubing.

Characteristics
- Numerous oscillations above and below baseline after activation of the fast-flush device

Interventions
- Examine the tubing and remove all air bubbles from the fluid system.

Troubleshooting the pressure monitoring system

Problem	Possible causes	Nursing interventions
No waveform	• Power supply turned off • Monitor screen pressure range set too low • Loose connection in line • Transducer not connected to amplifier • Stopcock off to patient • Catheter occluded or out of blood vessel	• Check the power supply. • Raise the monitor screen pressure range if necessary. • Rebalance and recalibrate the equipment. • Tighten loose connections. • Position the stopcock correctly. • Use the fast-flush valve to flush the line, or try to aspirate blood from the catheter. If the line remains blocked, notify the doctor and prepare to replace the line.
Drifting waveforms	• Improper warm-up • Electrical cable kinked or compressed • Temperature change in room air or IV flush solution	• Allow the monitor and transducer to warm up for 10 to 15 minutes. • Place the monitor's cable where it can't be stepped on or compressed. • Routinely zero and calibrate the equipment 30 minutes after setting it up to allow IV fluid to warm to room temperature.
Line fails to flush	• Stopcocks positioned incorrectly • Inadequate pressure from pressure bag • Kink in pressure tubing • Blood clot in catheter	• Make sure stopcocks are positioned correctly. • Make sure the pressure bag gauge reads 300 mm Hg. • Check the pressure tubing for kinks. • Try to aspirate the clot with a syringe. If the line still won't flush, notify the doctor and prepare to replace the line, if necessary. *Important:* Never use a syringe to flush a hemodynamic line.
Artifact (waveform interference)	• Patient movement • Electrical interference • Catheter fling (tip of pulmonary artery catheter moving rapidly in large blood vessel or heart chamber)	• Wait until the patient is quiet before taking a reading. • Make sure electrical equipment is connected and grounded correctly. • Notify the doctor, who may try to reposition the catheter.
False-high readings	• Transducer balancing port positioned below patient's right atrium • Flush solution flow rate is too fast • Air in system • Catheter fling (tip of pulmonary artery catheter moving rapidly in large blood vessel or heart chamber)	• Position the balancing port level with the patient's right atrium. • Check the flush solution flow rate. Maintain it at 3 to 4 mL/hr. • Remove air from the lines and the transducer. • Notify the doctor, who may try to reposition the catheter.

Problem	Possible causes	Nursing interventions
False-low readings	• Transducer balancing port positioned above right atrium • Transducer imbalance • Loose connection	• Position the balancing port level with the patient's right atrium. • Make sure the transducer's flow system isn't kinked or occluded, and rebalance and recalibrate the equipment. • Tighten loose connections.
Damped waveform	• Air bubbles • Blood clot in catheter • Blood flashback in line • Incorrect transducer position • Arterial catheter out of blood vessel or pressed against vessel wall	• Secure all connections. • Remove air from the lines and the transducer. • Check for and replace cracked equipment. • Refer to "Line fails to flush" (earlier in this chart). • Make sure stopcock positions are correct; tighten loose connections, and replace cracked equipment; flush the line with the fast-flush valve; replace the transducer dome if blood backs up into it. • Make sure the transducer is kept at the level of the right atrium at all times. Improper levels give false-high or false-low pressure readings. • Reposition the catheter if it's against the vessel wall. • Try to aspirate blood to confirm proper placement in the vessel. If you can't aspirate blood, notify the doctor and prepare to replace the line. *Note:* Bloody drainage at the insertion site may indicate catheter displacement. Notify the doctor immediately.

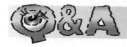

Identify the pieces of equipment in a pressure monitoring system indicated on this illustration.

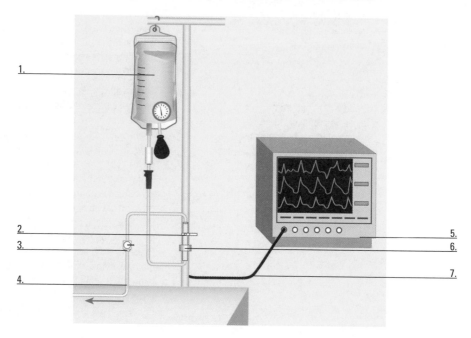

Match the following pressure monitoring problems with their causes:

1. No wave form _____   **A.** Air bubbles

2. Drifting waveform _____   **B.** Transducer imbalance

3. Lines fails to flush _____   **C.** Flush solution flow rate too fast

4. Artifact _____   **D.** Stopcocks positioned incorrectly

5. False-high readings _____   **E.** Electrical interference

6. False-low readings _____   **F.** Loose connection in line

7. Dampened waveform _____   **G.** Kinked electrical cable

Answers: Identify the pieces: Refer to pages 20-21. Match the following: 1. F, 2. G, 3. D, 4. E, 5. C, 6. B, 7. A.

Suggested References

Alspach, J.G. (Ed.). *Core Curriculum for Critical Care Nursing*, 6th ed. Philadelphia: W.B. Saunders Co., 2006.

Carlson, K.K. (Ed.). *AACN Advanced Critical Care Nursing*. Philadelphia: Elsevier, 2009.

Chulay, M., and Burns, S.M. *AACN Essentials of Critical Care Nursing*, 3rd ed. New York: McGraw-Hill, 2014.

Diepenbrock, N. *Quick Reference to Critical Care*, 4th ed. Philadelphia: Lippincott Williams & Wilkins, 2012.

Lippincott's Nursing Procedures & Skills. Philadelphia: Lippincott Williams & Wilkins, 2009. Accessed via the online program on September 1, 2009.

McLaughlin, M.A. (Ed.). *Cardiovascular Care Made Incredibly Easy*, 3rd ed. Philadelphia: Lippincott Williams & Wilkins, 2014.

Morton, P.G., and Fontaine, D.K. *Critical Care Nursing: A Holistic Approach*, 9th ed. Philadelphia: Lippincott Williams & Wilkins, 2009.

Chapter 3

Vascular access

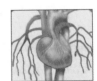

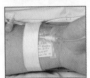

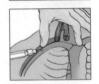

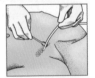

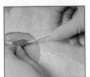

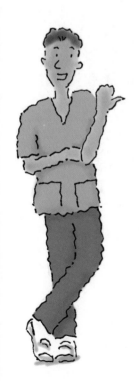

Arterial line insertion

A closer look at arterial insertion sites

Arterial line

An arterial line provides access for invasive arterial pressure monitoring (e.g., continuous blood pressure monitoring) and can be used to obtain blood samples when frequent blood draws are indicated, including arterial blood gases. Typically, a standard 18G to 20G over-the-needle catheter is inserted into a peripheral artery, usually the radial, brachial, or femoral artery. The radial artery is the preferred site.

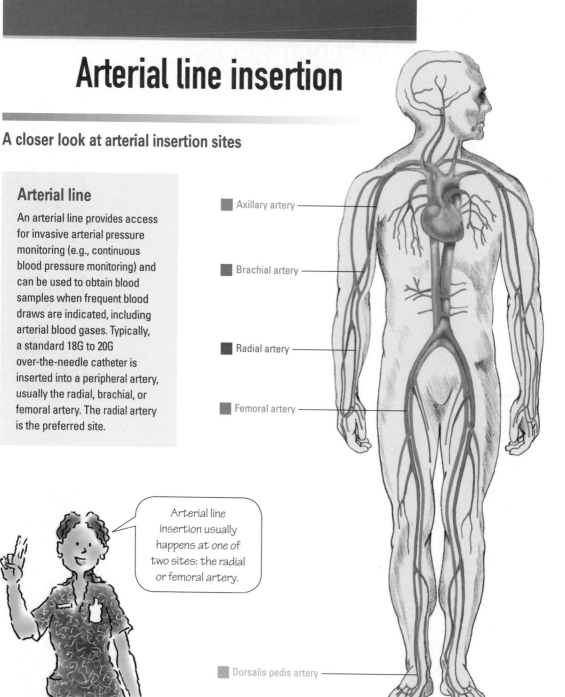

Axillary artery

Brachial artery

Radial artery

Femoral artery

Dorsalis pedis artery

Arterial line insertion usually happens at one of two sites: the radial or femoral artery.

Choosing an arterial catheter site

Let's make a list of all the pros and cons when it comes to choosing an arterial catheter site.

When your patient needs arterial pressure monitoring, an arterial catheter will probably be inserted in the radial artery. If these sites are unsuitable, the catheter may be inserted in the femoral, brachial, axillary, or dorsalis pedis artery. Regardless of the site chosen, the site should have an artery large enough to accommodate the arterial catheter without impeding distal blood flow to the site. It should also be free of infection or traumatic injury proximal to the insertion site.

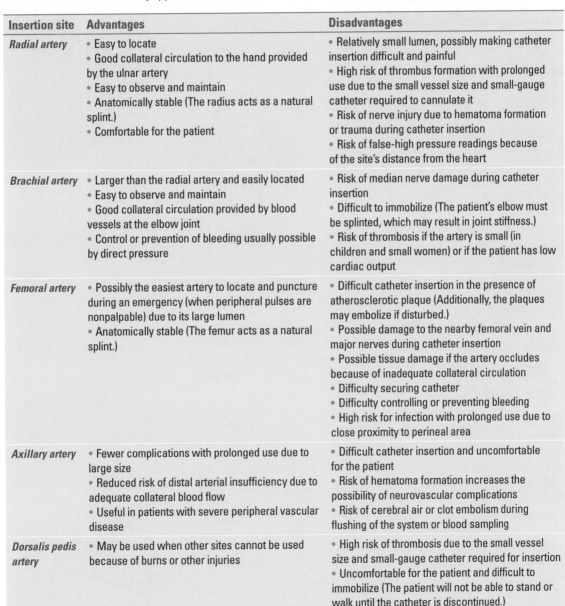

Insertion site	Advantages	Disadvantages
Radial artery	• Easy to locate • Good collateral circulation to the hand provided by the ulnar artery • Easy to observe and maintain • Anatomically stable (The radius acts as a natural splint.) • Comfortable for the patient	• Relatively small lumen, possibly making catheter insertion difficult and painful • High risk of thrombus formation with prolonged use due to the small vessel size and small-gauge catheter required to cannulate it • Risk of nerve injury due to hematoma formation or trauma during catheter insertion • Risk of false-high pressure readings because of the site's distance from the heart
Brachial artery	• Larger than the radial artery and easily located • Easy to observe and maintain • Good collateral circulation provided by blood vessels at the elbow joint • Control or prevention of bleeding usually possible by direct pressure	• Risk of median nerve damage during catheter insertion • Difficult to immobilize (The patient's elbow must be splinted, which may result in joint stiffness.) • Risk of thrombosis if the artery is small (in children and small women) or if the patient has low cardiac output
Femoral artery	• Possibly the easiest artery to locate and puncture during an emergency (when peripheral pulses are nonpalpable) due to its large lumen • Anatomically stable (The femur acts as a natural splint.)	• Difficult catheter insertion in the presence of atherosclerotic plaque (Additionally, the plaques may embolize if disturbed.) • Possible damage to the nearby femoral vein and major nerves during catheter insertion • Possible tissue damage if the artery occludes because of inadequate collateral circulation • Difficulty securing catheter • Difficulty controlling or preventing bleeding • High risk for infection with prolonged use due to close proximity to perineal area
Axillary artery	• Fewer complications with prolonged use due to large size • Reduced risk of distal arterial insufficiency due to adequate collateral blood flow • Useful in patients with severe peripheral vascular disease	• Difficult catheter insertion and uncomfortable for the patient • Risk of hematoma formation increases the possibility of neurovascular complications • Risk of cerebral air or clot embolism during flushing of the system or blood sampling
Dorsalis pedis artery	• May be used when other sites cannot be used because of burns or other injuries	• High risk of thrombosis due to the small vessel size and small-gauge catheter required for insertion • Uncomfortable for the patient and difficult to immobilize (The patient will not be able to stand or walk until the catheter is discontinued.)

Allen's test

Before accessing the radial artery for peripheral arterial line insertion, the patient's ulnar and radial circulation must be checked for collateral circulation. Why? If the radial artery is blocked by a blood clot (a common complication of arterial lines), the ulnar artery alone must supply blood to the hand. A simple, reliable test of circulation can be done by performing Allen's test, which demonstrates how well both arteries supply blood to the hand.

Remember: Use Allen's test to ensure that, if the radial artery is blocked, the ulnar artery will be able to supply blood to the hand.

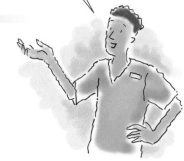

Steps for Performing the Allen's test

1 Rest the patient's arm on the mattress or bedside stand, and support his wrist with a rolled towel. Have him clench his fist. Then, using your index and middle fingers, press on the radial and ulnar arteries. Hold this position for a few seconds.

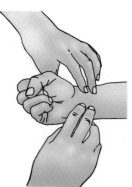

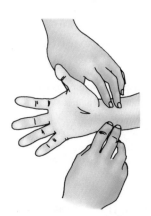

2 Without removing your fingers from the patient's arteries, ask him to unclench his fist and hold his hand in a relaxed position. The palm will be blanched because pressure from your fingers has impaired the normal blood flow.

3 Release pressure on the patient's ulnar artery but keep pressure on the radial artery, as shown at right. Observe the palm for a brisk return of color, which should occur within 7 seconds (showing a patent ulnar artery and adequate blood flow to the hand). If color returns in 7 to 15 seconds, blood flow is impaired; if color returns after 15 seconds, consider the flow inadequate.

   If blood flow is impaired or inadequate, the radial artery in this hand should not be used. At this point, proceed with Allen's test in the other hand. If neither hand colors, the brachial artery site may be considered for catheter insertion.

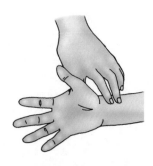

Caring for arterial catheters

There are three steps to basic care for arterial catheters:

1 dressing

2 immobilizing

3 assessing

Dressing

After insertion of the arterial catheter, dress the insertion site and change it according to facility policy. Sterile dressing changes are recommended. Transparent dressings are typically used over the insertion site because they enable complete visualization of the site. This breathable film allows oxygen in and moisture vapors out, while also providing barrier protection.

Immobilizing

The body part where the catheter is placed will then need to be immobilized. The joint or limb should be placed in a neutral position to prevent joint flexion or extension, which may result in kinking or dislodgment of the catheter. If the radial artery has been used, take care not to hyperextend the wrist, which could result in neuromuscular injury. Assess the limb for any associated pressure points when immobilizing the extremity. Regularly assess the functioning of arterial line to prevent kinking.

Assessing

The arterial catheter site must be assessed every hour. Include the following in your assessment:
• Inspect the arterial catheter insertion site for redness, drainage, bruising, or blanching. (The benefit of using a transparent dressing becomes apparent at this step.) Palpate the area for firmness or swelling.
• Assess circulation of the extremity in which the arterial catheter has been placed by evaluating skin color, temperature, capillary refill, distal pulses (if applicable), and motor and sensory function.

A closer look at an arterial line

This photo shows an arterial line taped in place in the radial artery. (Flush is shown in Chapter 4.)

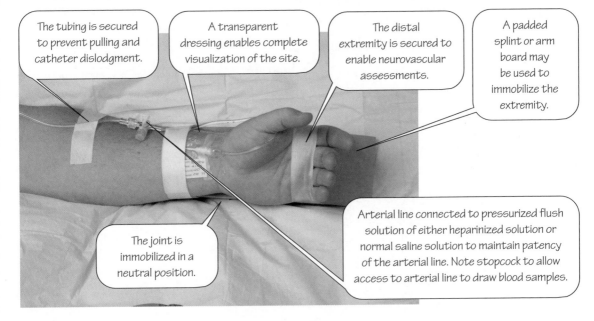

The tubing is secured to prevent pulling and catheter dislodgment.

A transparent dressing enables complete visualization of the site.

The distal extremity is secured to enable neurovascular assessments.

A padded splint or arm board may be used to immobilize the extremity.

The joint is immobilized in a neutral position.

Arterial line connected to pressurized flush solution of either heparinized solution or normal saline solution to maintain patency of the arterial line. Note stopcock to allow access to arterial line to draw blood samples.

CV and PA catheter insertion

CV and PA catheter insertion sites

The most common sites for percutaneous insertion of a central venous (CV) or pulmonary artery (PA) catheter include the internal jugular, subclavian, and femoral veins. The right internal jugular vein is considered the safest insertion site. Although the subclavian vein is easily accessed, its use carries certain risks. The most significant risk is pneumothorax, resulting from puncturing the lung at a level above the clavicle during catheter insertion. Additionally, using the subclavian vein may cause the catheter or the introducer to bend or kink during insertion. Although the femoral vein is easily accessible, use of this site carries an increased risk of infection due to the proximity to the groin.

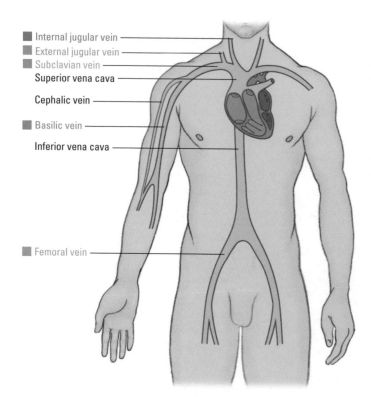

- Internal jugular vein
- External jugular vein
- Subclavian vein
Superior vena cava

Cephalic vein

- Basilic vein

Inferior vena cava

- Femoral vein

CV and PA catheterization

CV and PA catheterization can help you learn about a patient's cardiovascular and pulmonary status, obtain blood samples, and infuse solutions. Inserted in a surgical, sterile procedure in the jugular, subclavian, femoral, or basilic vein, the catheter is flow-directed, allowing venous circulation to carry it through to a position in or near the right atrium (for CV catheters) or through the right atrium and ventricle to the pulmonary artery (for PA catheters).

Choosing a CV or PA catheter insertion site

This chart highlights the advantages and disadvantages of the most common sites used for CV or PA catheter insertion. Catheter-related infection is the most common risk of every insertion site, occurring in up to 5% of cases.

Insertion site	Advantages	Disadvantages
Internal jugular vein	• Provides a short, direct route to the superior vena cava or right atrium • Carries a low risk of catheter displacement • Has a lower incidence of pneumothorax or perforation of an artery than with a subclavian vein • Has a lower risk of thrombotic complications because rapid infusion rates may be used	• Several possible complications, including: –air embolism –common carotid artery perforation –perforation of the trachea or endotracheal (ET) tube cuff –pneumothorax (more common in the left internal jugular vein) –injury to the thoracic duct (applicable only to left internal jugular vein)
External jugular vein (peripheral access)	• Is easily accessible due to its superficial location • Carries a low risk of pneumothorax or puncture of the carotid artery	• Difficult passage to the central veins • Increased risk of thrombosis because infusion rates must be slower • Difficulty maintaining a sterile dressing, especially with the presence of a tracheostomy • Several possible complications, including: –carotid artery perforation –pneumothorax –displacement into axillary vein
Subclavian vein	• Is easily accessible • Enables easy maintenance of a sterile, intact dressing • Allows the patient to move neck and arm freely • Carries minimal risk of catheter displacement after it is secured • Carries a reduced risk of thrombosis because rapid infusion rates are allowable	• Several possible complications, including: –air embolism –subclavian artery perforation –life-threatening blood loss (because pressure cannot be applied to an anterior subclavian tear) –pneumothorax –phrenic or brachial nerve injury –ET tube cuff perforation
Femoral vein	• Is easily accessible • Enables greater ease of insertion in patients with tortuous subclavian and jugular veins (such as in elderly patients) • Carries no risk of pneumothorax and a minimal risk of air embolism	• Possibly difficult to identify in obese patients • Increased risk of infection due to proximity to the groin • Difficulty maintaining a sterile, intact dressing • Increased risk of catheter displacement because the site is difficult to immobilize • Several possible complications, including: –inadvertent cannulation of local smaller veins –thrombosis
Basilic vein (peripheral access)	• Carries no risk of pneumothorax or major hemorrhage • Enables greater control in bleeding from the site	• Difficult to identify in obese or edematous patients • Possible difficulty advancing the catheter to the central veins from this distal site • Increased risk of catheter displacement • Several possible complications, including: –thrombosis –venous spasm

Insertion of the catheter

Prior to catheter insertion, assess the patient's vital signs, obtain consent and explain the procedure, and set up the appropriate tubing.

CV and PA catheters share the same approaches to insertion—a surgical cutdown technique or a percutaneous technique.

A *surgical cutdown* involves identifying the vein to be used for insertion, administering a local anesthetic, and making a small incision directly above the vessel. The catheter is then inserted by direct needle-puncture of the vessel, or by creating a tiny incision in the vessel, through which the catheter is inserted and then sutured in place. Surgical cutdown is typically performed for central catheters inserted through the basilic vein or when percutaneous access is not possible.

The more commonly used *percutaneous technique* involves the use of an introducer to access the vessel. A locator needle is first inserted in the vein, and a guide wire is threaded through the needle. The needle is removed, and an introducer catheter is inserted over the wire. Then the wire is removed, leaving the introducer in place in the blood vessel. The CV or PA catheter is then inserted through the introducer sheath. Prepackaged introducer kits are available to facilitate gathering and preparation of equipment, as shown below.

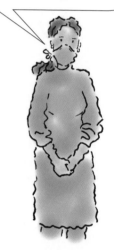

No matter which technique you use to insert a CV or PA catheter, it should be performed under strict sterile conditions.

Introducer kit

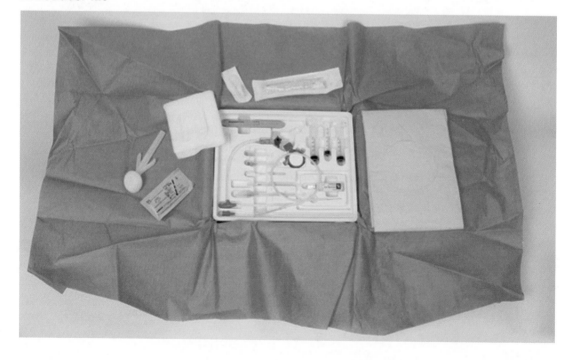

Patient positioning

Proper patient positioning during CV or PA catheter insertion is essential to enable optimal access to the site and prevent contamination. These guidelines will help you position your patient based on the insertion site you are using:

- Place the patient in Trendelenburg's position to dilate the veins and reduce the risk of air embolism. (This position is not necessary if you are using the femoral vein site.)
- For subclavian insertion, place a rolled blanket or towel lengthwise between the shoulders to increase venous distention.
- For jugular insertion, place a rolled blanket or towel under the opposite shoulder to extend the neck, making anatomic landmarks more visible.
- Turn the patient's head away from the site to prevent possible contamination from airborne pathogens and to make the site more accessible.
  - Other access sites may include femoral and antecubital veins.

Potential Complications during Insertion or after Placement

- Potential complications of a PA or central venous pressure (CVP) catheter during insertion may include pneumothorax, air embolism, arterial puncture, or bleeding. In addition, cardiac dysrhythmias may occur during PA catheter insertion. After-placement complications of CVP and PA catheters can include thrombosis and infection.

Positioning for subclavian vein access

In addition to placing a rolled blanket or towel lengthwise between the patient's shoulders, the patient should be positioned with her head turned away from the access site with the chin pointed upward, as shown here.

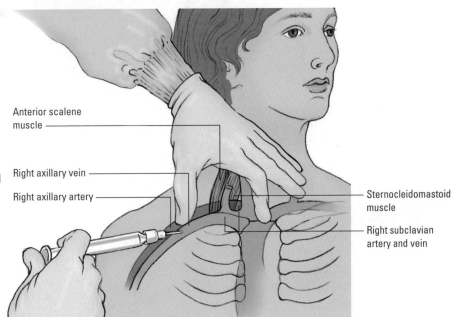

Anterior scalene muscle

Right axillary vein

Right axillary artery

Sternocleidomastoid muscle

Right subclavian artery and vein

A closer look at catheter insertion

These photos show a PA catheter being inserted through an introducer during a percutaneous insertion procedure.

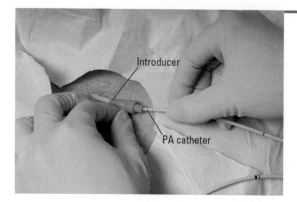

Introducer

PA catheter

1 After the introducer is in place, the PA catheter may be inserted.

2 Because the introducer completely occupies the puncture sites at the skin and blood vessel, there is minimal bleeding from the site.

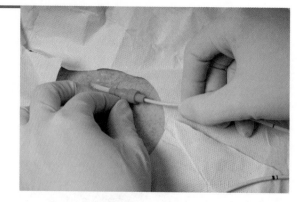

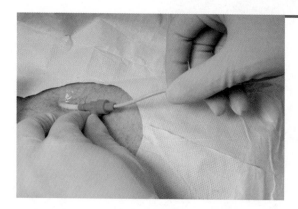

3 The PA catheter is inserted 5″ to 6″ to reach the superior vena cava from the internal jugular or right subclavian insertion sites. A longer length is required from the femoral site.

Key steps in changing a CV dressing

Expect to change your patient's CV dressing every 48 hours if it is a gauze dressing and at least every 7 days if it is transparent. Sterile dressing changes are indicated whenever the dressing becomes soiled, moist, or loose. These illustrations show the key steps you will perform.

First, put on a mask and clean gloves and remove the old dressing by pulling it toward the exit site of a long-term catheter or toward the insertion site of a short-term catheter. This technique helps you avoid pulling out the line. If a chlorhexidine disk is in place, remove it. Remove and discard your gloves.

Next, put on sterile gloves and clean the skin around the catheter with an antimicrobial skin cleanser (usually chlorhexidine), using a vigorous side-to-side motion (as shown below).

Allow the skin to dry completely. Apply a new chlorhexidine disk if indicated.

After the solution has dried, cover the site with a dressing, such as the transparent semipermeable dressing shown below. Write the time and date on the dressing.

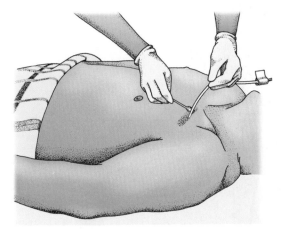 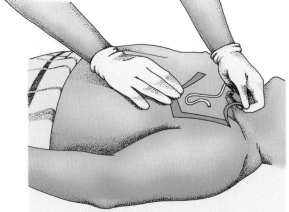

Indications for CVP or PA cathether

Both types of catheters can be very useful to evaluate volume status in acutely ill patients. The catheters can also be useful in determining if the patient has fluid-volume status changes and left ventricular heart dysfunction. The PA catheter can specifically provide continuous monitoring of the PA pressure and can be used to obtain a cardiac output. The pressure monitoring provided by the CVP or PA catheter can be useful in guiding the use of fluid therapy and/or vasoactive medication (e.g., dopamine) titration.

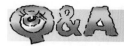

Able to label?

In the illustration, label the arterial insertion sites.

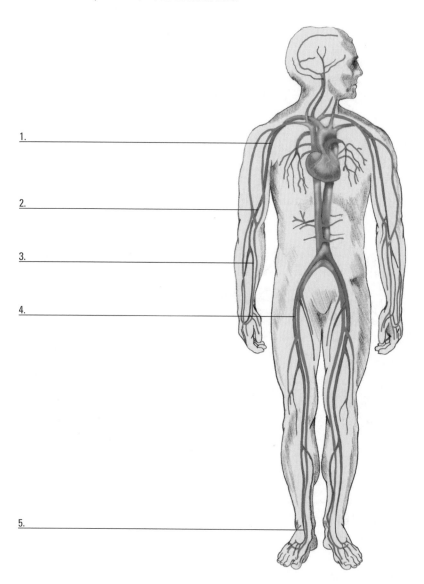

1. _____

2. _____

3. _____

4. _____

5. _____

True or false

1. An arterial line can measure CVP. True or False

2. Flush solutions used to maintain patency of arterial lines ALWAYS REQUIRE Heparin. True or False

3. Question: What action should you take as a nurse if the arterial line becomes disconnected from the tubing of the pressurized flush solution?

Answers: Able to label? 1. Axillary artery, 2. Brachial artery, 3. Radial artery, 4. Femoral artery, 5. Dorsal pedis artery. True or false: 1. FALSE, 2. FALSE, 3. Immediately apply pressure to arterial site to control bleeding.

Suggested References

Alspach, J.G. (Ed.). *Core Curriculum for Critical Care Nursing*, 6th ed. Philadelphia: W.B. Saunders Co., 2006.

McLaughlin, M.A. (Ed.). *Cardiovascular Care Made Incredibly Easy*, 3rd ed. Philadelphia: Lippincott Williams & Wilkins, 2014.

Carlson, K.K. (Ed.). *AACN Advanced Critical Care Nursing.* Philadelphia: Elsevier, 2009.

Chulay, M., and Burns, S.M. *AACN Essentials of Critical Care Nursing*, 3rd ed. New York: McGraw-Hill, 2014.

Diepenbrock, N. *Quick Reference to Critical Care*, 4th ed. Philadelphia: Lippincott Williams & Wilkins, 2012.

Lippincott's Nursing Procedures & Skills. Philadelphia: Lippincott Williams & Wilkins, 2009. Accessed via the online program on September 1, 2009.

Morton, P.G., and Fontaine, D.K. *Critical Care Nursing: A Holistic Approach*, 9th ed. Philadelphia: Lippincott Williams & Wilkins, 2009.

Scales, K., and Collie, E. "A Practical Guide to Using Pulmonary Artery Catheters," *Nursing Standard* 21(43):42–48, July 2007.

Weigand, D.L., and Carlson, K.K. *AACN Procedure Manual for Critical Care*, 6th ed. St. Louis: Elsevier Saunders, 2010.

Woods, S., et al. *Cardiac Nursing*, 6th ed. Philadelphia: Lippincott Williams & Wilkins, 2010.

Chapter 4

Arterial pressure monitoring

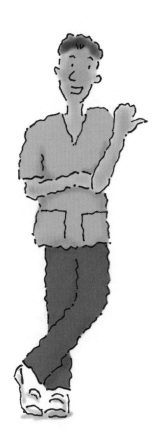

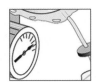

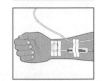

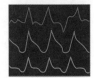

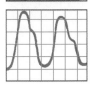

Arterial pressure monitoring basics

A closer look at an arterial pressure monitoring system

Arterial pressure monitoring

Arterial pressure monitoring measures arterial pressure directly, using an indwelling arterial catheter connected to an external pressure transducer and fluid-filled tubing. The tubing is attached to a pressure bag of saline or heparin flush solution and the transducer is attached to a monitor. The pressure transducer converts the pressure into an electrical signal that is interpreted and displayed on a monitor screen as a continuous waveform. The pressure may also be shown as a digital readout.

Most commonly, the radial artery is the site of catheter insertion because this artery is readily accessible. However, brachial or pedal artery may also be used.

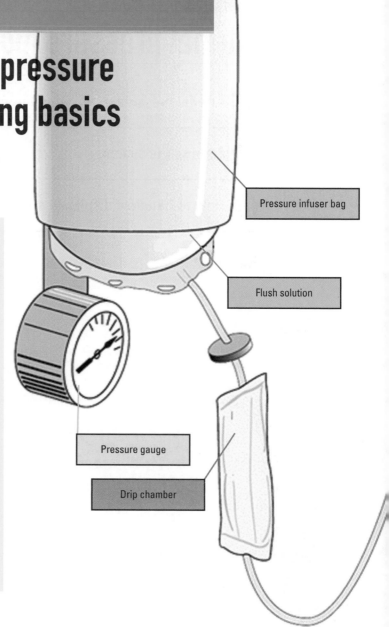

Pressure infuser bag

Flush solution

Pressure gauge

Drip chamber

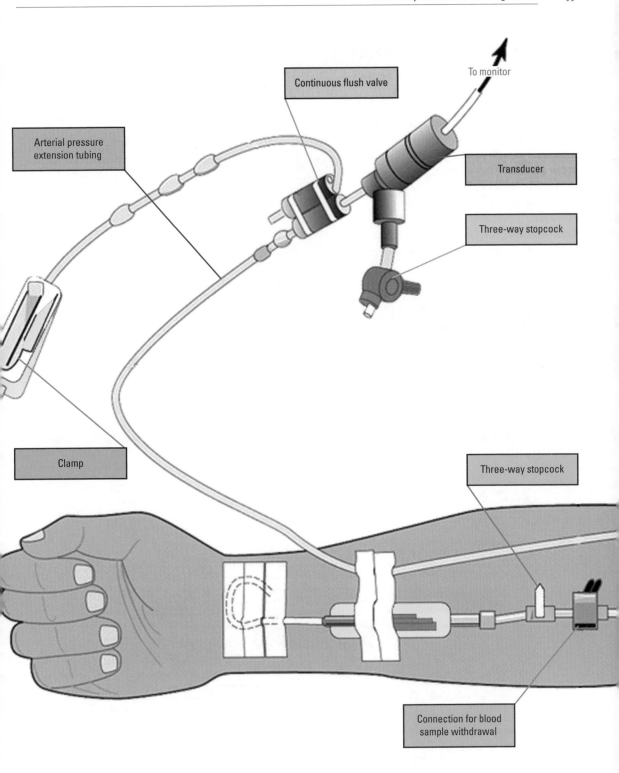

To monitor

Continuous flush valve

Transducer

Arterial pressure extension tubing

Three-way stopcock

Clamp

Three-way stopcock

Connection for blood sample withdrawal

Uses of arterial pressure monitoring

Direct arterial pressure monitoring permits continuous measurement of systolic, diastolic, and mean pressures and allows arterial blood sampling. Because direct measurement reflects systemic vascular resistance as well as blood flow, it is generally more accurate than indirect methods that are based on blood flow (such as palpation and auscultation for Korotkoff sounds). Moreover, direct arterial pressure monitoring aids in determining mean arterial pressure (MAP), an important indicator of tissue perfusion.

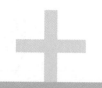

Indications

- When highly accurate or frequent blood pressure measurements are required
- For patients receiving doses of vasoactive drugs requiring titration
- For patients requiring frequent blood sampling

Contraindications

- Peripheral vascular disease
- Hemorrhagic disorders
- Use of anticoagulants or thrombolytic agents

Insertion site contraindications
- Areas of active infection or with synthetic graft materials
- Sites of prior vascular surgery

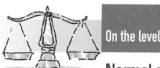

On the level

Normal arterial pressure parameters

In general, arterial systolic pressure reflects the peak pressure generated by the left ventricle. It also indicates compliance of the large arteries, or the *peripheral resistance.*

Arterial diastolic pressure reflects the runoff velocity and elasticity of the arterial system, particularly the arterioles.

MAP is the average pressure in the arterial system during systole and diastole. It reflects the driving, or *perfusion,* pressure and is determined by arterial blood volume and blood vessel elasticity and resistance. To compute MAP, use this formula:

$$MAP = \frac{systolic\ pressure + 2\ (diastolic\ pressure)}{3}$$

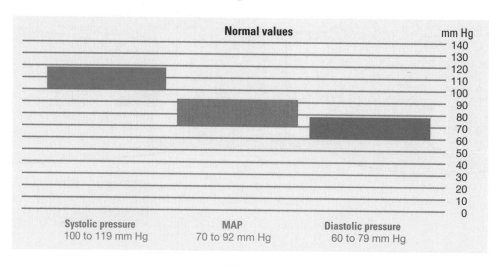

Normal values

mm Hg

Systolic pressure
100 to 119 mm Hg

MAP
70 to 92 mm Hg

Diastolic pressure
60 to 79 mm Hg

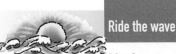

Understanding an arterial waveform

Normal arterial blood pressure produces a characteristic waveform representing ventricular systole and diastole. The waveform has five distinct components:

- anacrotic limb
- systolic peak
- dicrotic limb
- dicrotic notch
- end-diastole.

The anacrotic limb marks the waveform's initial upstroke, which results as blood is rapidly ejected from the ventricle through the open aortic valve into the aorta. The rapid ejection causes a sharp rise in arterial pressure, which appears as the waveform's highest point. This point is called the *systolic peak.*

As blood continues into the peripheral vessels, arterial pressure falls and the waveform begins a downward trend. This part is called the *dicrotic limb.* Arterial pressure usually continues to fall until pressure in the ventricle is less than pressure in the aortic root. When this unequal pressure occurs, the aortic valve closes. This event appears as a small notch on the waveform's downside, known as the *dicrotic notch.*

When the aortic valve closes, diastole begins, progressing until the aortic root pressure gradually descends to its lowest point. On the waveform, this is known as *end-diastole.*

> Knowing the components of an arterial waveform keeps you ahead of the wave on arterial pressure monitoring.

Normal arterial waveform

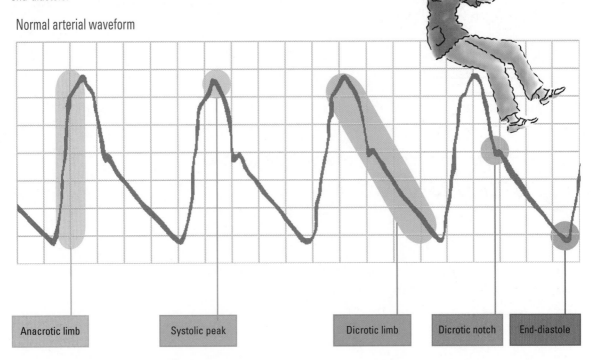

| Anacrotic limb | Systolic peak | Dicrotic limb | Dicrotic notch | End-diastole |

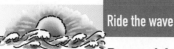

Ride the wave

Recognizing abnormal arterial waveforms

Understanding a normal arterial waveform is relatively straightforward. Unfortunately, an abnormal waveform is not so easy to decipher. Abnormal patterns and markings, however, may provide important diagnostic clues to the patient's cardiovascular status, or they may simply signal trouble in the monitor. Use this chart to help you recognize and resolve waveform abnormalities.

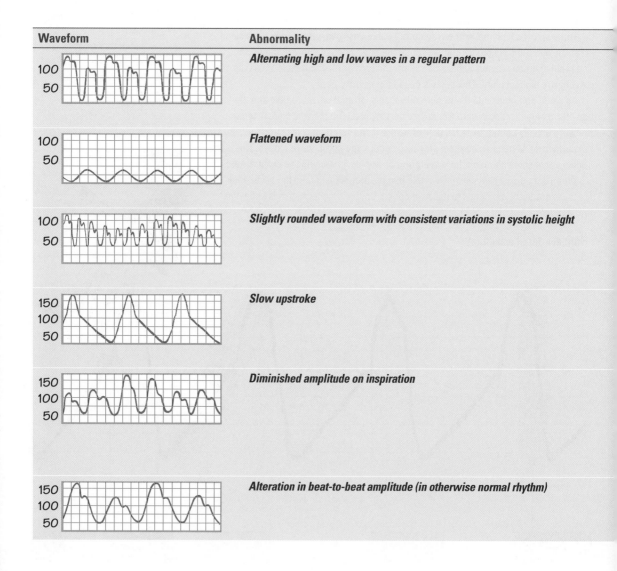

Waveform	Abnormality
	Alternating high and low waves in a regular pattern
	Flattened waveform
	Slightly rounded waveform with consistent variations in systolic height
	Slow upstroke
	Diminished amplitude on inspiration
	Alteration in beat-to-beat amplitude (in otherwise normal rhythm)

Possible causes	Nursing interventions
• Ventricular bigeminy	• Check the patient's ECG to confirm ventricular bigeminy. The tracing should reflect premature ventricular contractions every second beat.
• Overdamped waveform or hypotensive patient	• Check the patient's blood pressure with a sphygmomanometer. If you obtain a higher reading, suspect overdamping. Correct the problem by trying to aspirate the arterial line. If you succeed, flush the line. If the reading is very low or absent, suspect hypotension.
• Patient on ventilator with positive end-expiratory pressure	• Check the patient's systolic blood pressure regularly. The difference between the highest and lowest systolic pressure reading should be less than 10 mm Hg. If the difference exceeds that amount, suspect pulsus paradoxus, possibly from cardiac tamponade.
• Aortic stenosis	• Check the patient's heart sounds for signs of aortic stenosis. Also notify the doctor, who will document suspected aortic stenosis in his notes.
• Pulsus paradoxus, possibly from cardiac tamponade, constrictive pericarditis, or lung disease	• Note systolic pressure during inspiration and expiration. If inspiratory pressure is at least 10 mm Hg less than expiratory pressure, call the doctor. • If you are also monitoring pulmonary artery pressure, observe for a diastolic plateau. This abnormality occurs when the mean central venous pressure (right atrial pressure), mean pulmonary artery pressure, and mean pulmonary artery wedge pressure (pulmonary artery obstructive pressure) are within 5 mm Hg of one another.
• Pulsus alternans, which may indicate left ventricular failure	• Observe the patient's ECG, noting any deviation in the waveform. • Notify the doctor if this is a new and sudden abnormality.

Zeroing the system

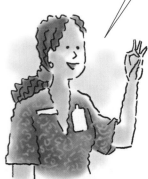

When it comes to accurate arterial pressure monitoring, zero is the magic number!

Because it is fluid-filled, an arterial pressure monitoring system must be zeroed. Remember that zeroing balances the transducer to atmospheric pressure, so that it reads 0 mm Hg when open to air. The procedure for zeroing the monitoring system is described fully in Chapter 2. These photos highlight some of the key steps in the procedure as it is performed on a peripheral arterial line.

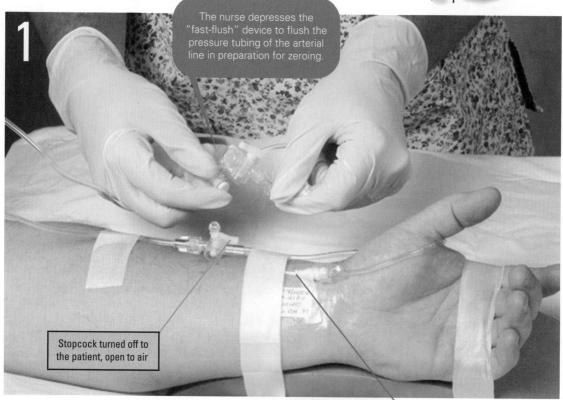

1

The nurse depresses the "fast-flush" device to flush the pressure tubing of the arterial line in preparation for zeroing.

Stopcock turned off to the patient, open to air

Arterial catheter insertion site

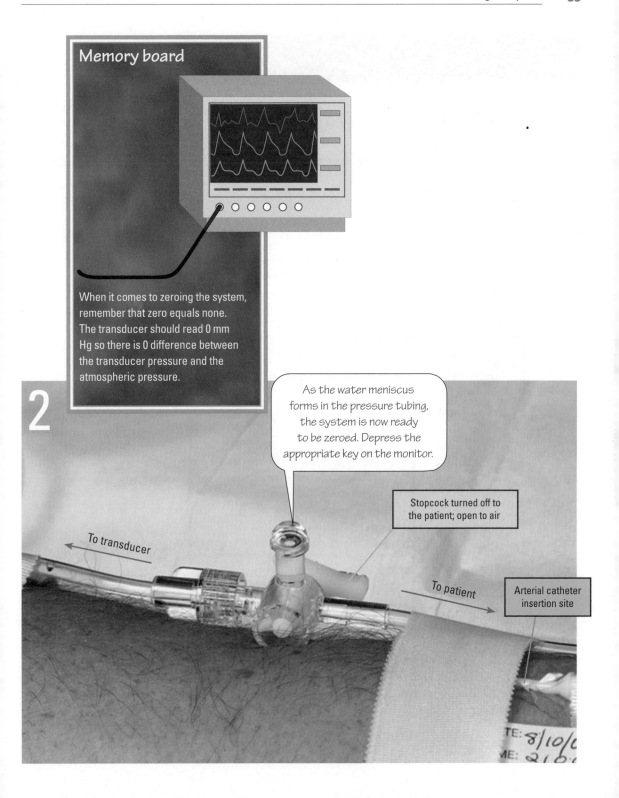

Memory board

When it comes to zeroing the system, remember that zero equals none. The transducer should read 0 mm Hg so there is 0 difference between the transducer pressure and the atmospheric pressure.

2

As the water meniscus forms in the pressure tubing, the system is now ready to be zeroed. Depress the appropriate key on the monitor.

Stopcock turned off to the patient; open to air

To transducer

To patient

Arterial catheter insertion site

TE: 8/10/0
ME: 21.0

How to handle a displaced arterial line

Your patient is in danger of hypovolemic shock from blood loss if his arterial line is pulled out or otherwise displaced.

After the bleeding stops

7 Withdraw blood for a complete blood count and arterial blood gas analysis, as ordered.

6 Assist the doctor as he inserts another catheter. Make sure that the patient's arm is immobilized and that the tubing and catheter are secure.

5 Estimate the amount of blood loss from your observations of the blood and from the changes in the patient's blood pressure and heart rate.

3 Apply a sterile pressure dressing.

4 Reassess the patient's level of consciousness (LOC) and orientation, and offer reassurance.

2 Check the patient's IV line and, if ordered, increase the flow rate temporarily to compensate for blood loss.

What to do first

1 Immediately apply direct pressure at the insertion site, and have someone summon the doctor. Because arterial blood flows under high intravascular pressure, be certain to maintain firm, direct pressure for a minimum of 5 minutes to encourage clot formation at the insertion site.

Ongoing care

Frequently assess the patient's vital signs, LOC, skin color and temperature, and circulation at the insertion site and beyond.

Watch for further bleeding or hematoma formation at the insertion site.

When the patient's condition stabilizes, reduce the IV flow rate to the previous keep-vein-open level.

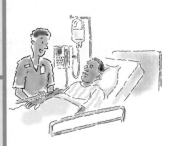

Minimizing complications of arterial pressure monitoring

For most critically ill patients, the advantages of arterial lines outweigh the disadvantages. However, because any invasive hemodynamic monitoring procedure poses some risk, you will need to watch your patient for complications that may result from an arterial line.

Complications and signs and symptoms	Possible causes	Nursing interventions	Prevention
Thrombosis • Loss or weakening of pulse below arterial line insertion site • Loss of warmth, sensation, color, and mobility in limb below insertion site • Damped or straight waveform on monitor display or printout	• Arterial damage during or after insertion • Sluggish flow rate of flush solution • Failure to heparinize flush solution adequately • Failure to flush catheter routinely and after withdrawing blood samples • Irrigation of clotted catheter with a syringe	• Notify the doctor. He may remove the line. • Document the complication and record your interventions.	• Check the patient's pulse rate immediately after catheter insertion, then once hourly. • Reduce injury to the artery by splinting the limb holding the line and by taping the catheter securely. • Check the flush solution's flow rate hourly; maintain the rate at 3 to 4 mL/hr. • Check the pressure infuser bag to make sure that pressure is maintained at 300 mm Hg. • Heparinize the flush solution according to facility policy. • Flush the catheter once hourly and after withdrawing blood samples. • Never irrigate an arterial catheter. You may flush a blood clot into the bloodstream.

Continued...

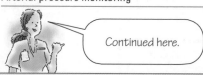

Continued here.

Complications and signs and symptoms	Possible causes	Nursing interventions	Prevention
Blood loss • Bloody dressing; blood flowing from disconnected line	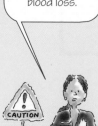 A dislodged catheter or disconnected line could cause blood loss.	• Stop the bleeding. • Check the patient's vital signs. • Notify the doctor if blood loss is great or if the patient's vital signs change. • If the line is disconnected, avoid reconnecting it. Instead, immediately replace contaminated equipment. • If the catheter is pulled out of the artery, remove it and apply direct pressure to the site; then notify the doctor. • When the bleeding stops, check the patient's pulse and the insertion site frequently for signs of thrombosis or hematoma. • Document the complication and record your interventions.	• Check the line connections and insertion site frequently. • Tape the catheter securely and splint the patient's limb. • Make sure that the monitor alarms are enabled.
Air embolism or thromboembolism • Drop in blood pressure • Rise in central venous pressure • Weak, rapid pulse • Cyanosis • Loss of consciousness • Damped waveform	• Air in tubing • Loose connections	• Place the patient on his left side and in Trendelenburg's position. If air has entered the heart chambers, this position may keep the air on the heart's right side. The pulmonary artery can then absorb the small air bubbles. • Check the arterial line for leaks. • Notify the doctor immediately, and check the patient's vital signs. • Administer oxygen if ordered. • Document the complication and record your interventions.	• Expel all air from the line before connecting it to the patient. • Make sure that all connections are secure; then check connections routinely. • Change the flush solution bag before it empties. • Prevent thromboembolism by keeping the arterial line patent with heparin flush solution.
Systemic infection • Sudden rise in temperature and pulse rate • Chills and shaking • Blood pressure changes	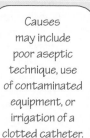 Causes may include poor aseptic technique, use of contaminated equipment, or irrigation of a clotted catheter.	• Look for other sources of infection first. Obtain urine, sputum, and blood specimens for cultures and other analyses, as ordered. • Notify the doctor. He may discontinue the line and send the equipment to the laboratory for study. • Document the complication and record your interventions.	• Review care procedures and ensure sterile technique. • Take care not to contaminate the arterial line insertion site when bathing the patient. • If any part of the line disconnects accidentally, do not rejoin it. Instead, replace the parts with sterile equipment. • Change system components as recommended (IV flush solution and pressure tubing every 96 hours, transparent dressing every 7 days, and nontransparent dressing every 24 to 48 hours).

Complications and signs and symptoms	Possible causes	Nursing interventions	Prevention
Arterial spasm • Intermittent loss or weakening of pulse below insertion site • Irregular waveform on monitor screen or printout	• Trauma to vessel during catheter insertion • Artery irritated by catheter after insertion	• Notify the doctor. • Prepare lidocaine (Xylocaine), which the doctor may inject directly into the arterial catheter to relieve the spasm. *Caution:* Make sure that a combination product containing lidocaine and epinephrine (Xylocaine with Epinephrine) is not used; the epinephrine in this product could cause further arterial constriction. • Document the complication and record your interventions.	• Tape the catheter securely to prevent it from moving in the artery. • Splint the patient's limb to stabilize the catheter.
Hematoma • Swelling at insertion site and generalized swelling of limb holding arterial line • Bleeding at site	• Blood leakage around catheter (resulting from weakened or damaged artery) • Failure to maintain pressure at site after removing catheter	• Stop the bleeding. • If the hematoma appears while the catheter is in place, notify the doctor. • If the hematoma appears within 30 minutes after you remove the catheter, apply ice to the site. Otherwise, apply warm, moist compresses to help speed the hematoma's absorption. • Document the complication and record your interventions.	• Tape the catheter securely and splint the insertion area to prevent damage to the artery. • After the catheter is removed, apply firm, manual pressure over the site for a minimum of 5 minutes or until bleeding stops.
Inaccurate pressure readings	*False-high values* • Transducer positioned too low • Small air bubbles in arterial line *False-low values* • Transducer positioned too high • Large air bubble in arterial line	• Relevel and rezero the transducer system. • Remove air bubbles. • Relevel and rezero the transducer system. • Remove air bubble. • Document the complication and record your interventions.	• Make sure to zero and calibrate the transducer system precisely. • Properly level the transducer at the level of the patient's right atrium (the phlebostatic axis). • Keep air from entering the pressure tubing or system. • Check the arterial waveform configuration for abnormalities.

What's a sure sign of inaccurate pressure readings? Your patient's clinical appearance is inconsistent with pressure values.

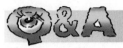

List six complications of arterial pressure monitoring:

1. _____

2. _____

3. _____

4. _____

5. _____

6. _____

Answers: Thrombosis, Blood loss, Embolism, Hematoma, Arterial spasm, Systemic infection.

Matchmaker

Match the abnormal arterial waveforms in column 2 to their descriptions in column 1.

Question: Inaccurate pressure readings could be caused by an air bubble in what line?

Answer: _____

1. Alternating high and low waves in a regular pattern _____   A.

2. Flattened waveform _____   B.

3. Slightly rounded waveform with consistent variations in systolic height _____   C.

4. Slow upstroke _____   D.

5. Diminished amplitude on inspiration _____   E.

6. Alteration in beat-to-beat amplitude (in otherwise normal rhythm) _____

F.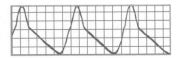

Answers: Question: Arterial. Matchmaker: 1. B, 2. D, 3. A, 4. F, 5. C, 6. E.

Suggested References

Alspach, J.G. (Ed.). *Core Curriculum for Critical Care Nursing*, 6th ed. Philadelphia: W.B. Saunders Co., 2006.

Carlson, K.K. (Ed.). *AACN Advanced Critical Care Nursing*. Philadelphia: Elsevier, 2009.

Chulay, M., and Burns, S.M. *AACN Essentials of Critical Care Nursing*, 3rd ed. New York: McGraw-Hill, 2014.

Diepenbrock, N. *Quick Reference to Critical Care*, 4th ed. Philadelphia: Lippincott Williams & Wilkins, 2012.

Lippincott's Nursing Procedures & Skills. Philadelphia: Lippincott Williams & Wilkins, 2009. Accessed via the online program on September 1, 2009.

McLaughlin, M.A. (Ed.). *Cardiovascular Care Made Incredibly Easy*, 3rd ed. Philadelphia: Lippincott Williams & Wilkins, 2014

Morton, P.G., and Fontaine, D.K. *Critical Care Nursing: A Holistic Approach*, 9th ed. Philadelphia: Lippincott Williams & Wilkins, 2009.

O'Grady, N.P., et al. Centers for Disease Control. 2011 Guidelines for the Prevention of Intravascular Catheter-Related Infections, 2011. Accessed from http://www.cdc.gov/hicpac/BSI/02-bsi-summary-of-recommendations-2011.html on November 14, 2014.

Scales, K., and Collie, E. "A Practical Guide to Using Pulmonary Artery Catheters," *Nursing Standard* 21(43):42–48, July 2007.

Weigand, D.L., and Carlson, K.K. *AACN Procedure Manual for Critical Care*, 6th ed. St. Louis: Elsevier Saunders, 2010.

Woods, S., et al. *Cardiac Nursing*, 6th ed. Philadelphia: Lippincott Williams & Wilkins, 2010.

Chapter 5

Central venous pressure monitoring

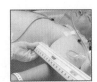

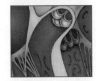

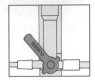

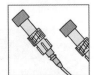

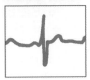

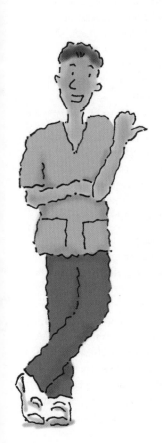

CVP monitoring

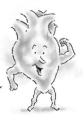

CVP helps indirectly gauge how well I'm pumping.

A closer look at a CV catheter

Clamps

Clamps prevent the backflow of blood or inadvertent administration of fluid through lumens that aren't in use.

Winged hub

The winged hub may be used to suture the catheter in place and provide improved stability when securing and dressing the insertion site.

Measurement markers

Measurement markers along the catheter aid in catheter insertion.

Antiseptic surface

Some catheters have an antiseptic coating of silver-sulfadiazine and chlorhexidine that may help reduce the incidence of catheter-associated infection.

Central venous pressure monitoring

In central venous pressure (CVP) monitoring, the physician or licensed independent provider inserts a catheter through a vein and advances it until its tip lies in or near the right atrium. Because no major valves lie at the junction of the vena cava and right atrium, pressure at end-diastole reflects back to the catheter. When connected to a transducer or manometer, the catheter measures CVP, a direct reflection of right atrial pressure and an indirect measure of preload of the right ventricle.

What it does

CVP monitoring helps to assess cardiac function, evaluate venous return to the heart, and the volume status of the body. The central venous (CV) line also provides access to a large vessel for rapid, high-volume fluid administration and enables frequent blood withdrawal for laboratory samples.

Intermittent or continuous?

CVP monitoring can be done intermittently or continuously. Typically, a single lumen CVP line is used for intermittent pressure readings using a disposable plastic water manometer. CVP is recorded in centimeters of water (cm H_2O) or millimeters of mercury (mm Hg) read from manometer markings. However, more commonly, a pressure transducer system is used to measure continuous CVP. A single CVP pressure carries little significance. It is the trend of the values that is more important to the clinical picture.

Obtaining CVP measurements

1 Make sure that the CV line or the proximal lumen of a pulmonary artery catheter is attached to the system. (If the patient has a CV line with multiple lumens, one lumen may be dedicated to continuous CVP monitoring and the other lumens used for fluid administration.)

2 Set up a pressure transducer system. Connect nonpliable pressure tubing from the CVP catheter hub to the transducer. Then connect the flush solution container to a flush device.

3 To obtain values, position the patient flat. If he cannot tolerate this position, elevate the bed to 30 degrees. Locate the level of the right atrium by identifying the phlebostatic axis. Zero the transducer, leveling the transducer air–fluid interface stopcock with the right atrium, as shown in the photo above right. Read the CVP value from the digital display on the monitor, and note the waveform. Make sure that the patient is still when the reading is taken to prevent artifact. Use this position (flat or 30 degrees) for all subsequent readings and when zeroing the transducer.

4 Intrathoracic pressure varies with respiration, affecting the CVP value. The best point in time at which to measure the CVP is at end-expiration, when intrathoracic pressure is closest to atmospheric pressure.

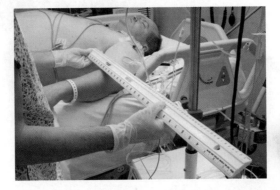

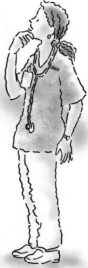

Correlating CVP with cardiac function

Essentially, CVP measurements reflect events in the cardiac cycle, and thus depict cardiac function.

> During ventricular diastole, the atrioventricular (AV) valves open.

> As diastole ends, each open valve creates what amounts to a common heart chamber.

> The pressure created by blood volume in the ventricles then extends back into the atria so that pressure measured in the right atrium indirectly mirrors the volume status of the right ventricle (called *preload*).

> During systole, the AV valves close and the semilunar valves open.

> At this point, the pressure measured in the atria indicates atrial filling.

CV catheter pathways

These illustrations show several common pathways for CV catheter insertion. Typically, a CV catheter is inserted in the subclavian or internal jugular vein.

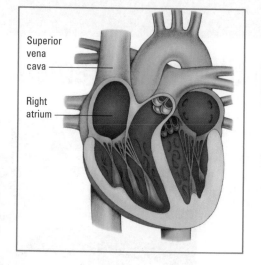

Superior vena cava

Right atrium

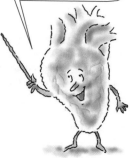

A CV catheter usually ends in the superior vena cava. However, it can also terminate in the right atrium.

Catheter

Insertion
- Subclavian vein

Termination
- Superior vena cava

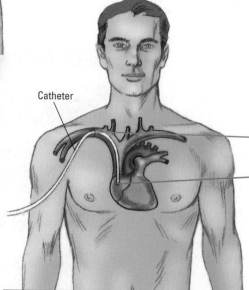

Catheter

Insertion
- Subclavian vein

Termination
- Right atrium

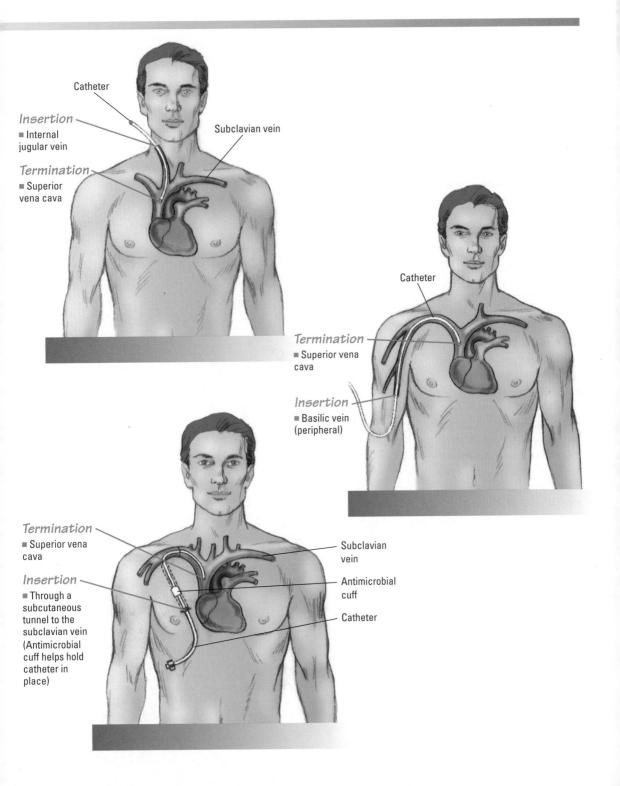

Catheter

Insertion
- Internal jugular vein

Termination
- Superior vena cava

Subclavian vein

Catheter

Termination
- Superior vena cava

Insertion
- Basilic vein (peripheral)

Termination
- Superior vena cava

Insertion
- Through a subcutaneous tunnel to the subclavian vein (Antimicrobial cuff helps hold catheter in place)

Subclavian vein

Antimicrobial cuff

Catheter

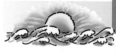

Ride the wave

Understanding the CVP waveform

When the CV catheter is attached to a pressure monitoring system, the bedside monitor can usually display digital pressure values, CVP waveforms, and ECG tracings. Synchronizing the CVP waveform with the ECG helps you identify components of the tracing. Keep in mind that cardiac electrical activity precedes the mechanical activities of systole and diastole.

Comparing electrical activity

The **P** wave on the ECG reflects atrial depolarization, which is then followed by atrial contraction and increased atrial pressure. Corresponding to the PR interval on the ECG, the **a** wave sequence on the CVP waveform represents atrial contraction.

The **x** descent on the CVP waveform represents atrial relaxation and declining pressure after systole, when the atrium expels blood into the ventricle.

As the cardiac cycle progresses, the tricuspid valve closes, producing a small backward bulge known as the **c** *wave.*

The atrium filling with venous blood during diastole produces another rise in pressure and a **v** wave, which corresponds to the **T** wave of the ECG.

After atrial filling, the tricuspid valve opens. Most of the blood in the right atrium passively empties into the right ventricle, causing atrial pressure to fall. On the CVP waveform, this decline appears as the **y** descent.

The **a** and **v** waves are almost the same height, indicating that atrial systole and atrial diastole produce about the same amount of pressure. Consequently, right atrial pressures are recorded as mean values because they are almost the same.

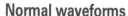

Normal waveforms

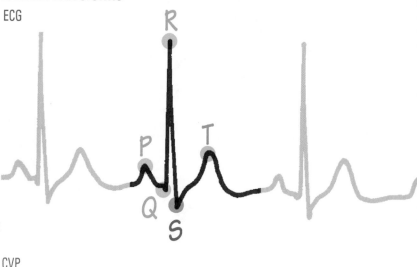

Synchronizing the CVP waveform with the ECG helps identify components. Keep in mind that cardiac electrical activity precedes systole and diastole.

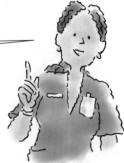

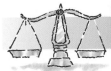

On the level

Normal CVP Values

CVP or right atrial pressure shows right ventricular function and end-diastolic pressure.

Causes of increased pressure

- Right-sided heart failure
- Volume overload
- Tricuspid valve stenosis or insufficiency
- Constrictive pericarditis
- Pulmonary hypertension
- Cardiac tamponade
- Right ventricular infarction

Normal values

Normal mean pressure ranges from 2 to 6 mm Hg (3 to 8 cm H_2O).

Causes of decreased pressure

- Reduced circulating blood volume

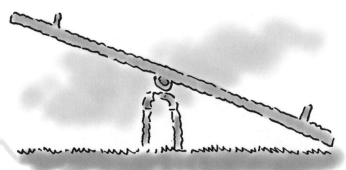

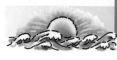

Recognizing abnormal CVP waveforms

Elevated a wave

ECG

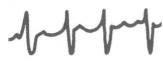

CVP

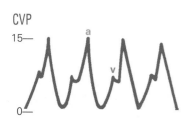

Physiologic causes
- Increased resistance to ventricular filling
- Increased atrial contraction

Associated conditions
- Heart failure
- Tricuspid stenosis
- Pulmonary hypertension

Elevated v wave

ECG

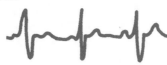

CVP

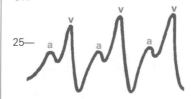

Physiologic cause
- Regurgitant flow

Associated conditions
- Tricuspid insufficiency
- Inadequate closure of the tricuspid valve due to heart failure

Absent a wave

ECG

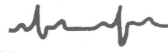

CVP

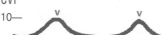

Physiologic cause
- Decreased or absent atrial contraction

Associated conditions
- Atrial fibrillation
- Junctional arrhythmias
- Ventricular pacing

Elevated a and v waves

CVP

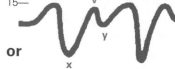

or

CVP

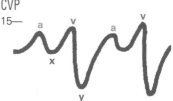

Physiologic causes
- Increased resistance to ventricular filling, which causes an elevated a wave
- Functional regurgitation, which causes an elevated v wave

Associated conditions
- Cardiac tamponade (smaller y descent than x descent)
- Constrictive pericardial disease (y descent exceeds x descent)
- Heart failure
- Hypervolemia
- Atrial hypertrophy

Measuring CVP with a water manometer

To ensure accurate CVP readings, make sure that the manometer base is aligned with the patient's right atrium (the zero reference point). The manometer set usually contains a leveling rod to allow you to determine this alignment quickly.

After adjusting the manometer's position, examine the three-way stopcock. By turning it to any position shown below, you can control the direction of fluid flow. Four-way stopcocks are also available.

All openings blocked

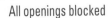

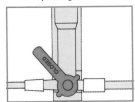

Manometer to patient   IV solution to manometer

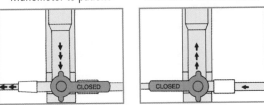

IV solution to patient

Converting pressure values

Although most facilities today use the pressure transducer system to measure CVP, the water manometer—the first device developed for monitoring CVP—may still be in use in some facilities. Both methods measure right atrial pressure—the pressure transducer in mm Hg and the water manometer in cm H_2O. If your facility uses both pressure transducers and water manometers, you may have to convert pressure values.

Use this formula to convert cm H_2O to mm Hg:

$$cm\ H_2O \div 1.36 = mm\ Hg$$

Conversely, use this formula to change mm Hg to cm H_2O:

$$mm\ Hg \times 1.36 = mm\ H_2O$$

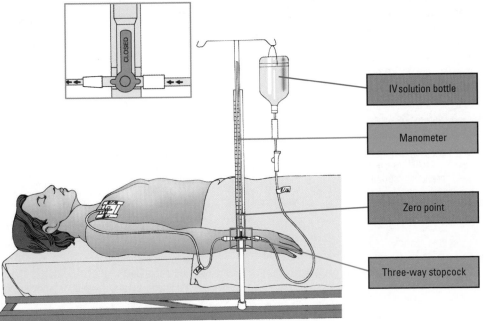

IV solution bottle

Manometer

Zero point

Three-way stopcock

Minimizing complications of CVP monitoring

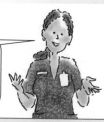

Many complications of CVP monitoring can be minimized with the right nursing interventions.

Problem	Signs and symptoms	Possible causes
Infection	• Redness, warmth, tenderness, swelling at insertion or exit site • Possible exudate of purulent material • Local rash or pustules • Fever, chills, malaise • Leukocytosis	• Failure to maintain sterile technique during catheter insertion or care • Wet or soiled dressing remaining on site • Immunosuppression • Contaminated catheter or solution • Frequent opening of catheter or long-term use of single IV access site • Failure to use good antiseptic technique when accessing the IV port
Pneumothorax, hemothorax, chylothorax, hydrothorax	• Decreased breath sounds on affected side • With hemothorax, decreased hemoglobin level because of blood pooling • Abnormal chest X-ray	• Repeated or long-term use of same vein • Preexisting cardiovascular disease • Lung puncture by catheter during insertion or exchange over a guide wire • Large blood vessel puncture with bleeding inside or outside the lung • Lymph node puncture with leakage of lymph fluid • Infusion of solution into chest area through infiltrated catheter
Air embolism	• Respiratory distress • Unequal breath sounds • Weak pulse • Increased CV pressure • Decreased blood pressure • Alteration or loss of consciousness	• Intake of air into the CV system during catheter insertion or tubing changes, or inadvertent opening, cutting, or breaking of catheter
Thrombosis	• Edema at puncture site • Erythema • Ipsilateral swelling of arm, neck, and face • Pain along vein • Fever, malaise • Chest pain • Dyspnea • Cyanosis	• Sluggish flow rate • Composition of catheter material (PVC catheters are more thrombogenic.) • Hypercoagulable state of patient • Preexisting limb edema • Infusion of irritating solutions

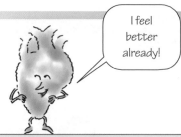

I feel better already!

Nursing interventions	Prevention
• Monitor vital signs closely. • Re-dress the site using sterile technique. • Use a chlorhexidine-impregnated sponge at the insertion site. • Treat systemically with antibiotics or antifungals, depending on culture results. • Catheter may be removed. • Draw central and peripheral blood cultures; if the same organism appears in both, then the catheter is the primary source and should be removed. • If cultures do not match but are positive, the catheter may be removed or the infection may be treated through the catheter. • If the catheter is removed, culture its tip per facility policy. • Document interventions.	• Maintain sterile technique. Use sterile gloves, masks, and gowns when appropriate. • Clean the port per facility policy before injecting or withdrawing. • Observe dressing-change protocols. • Change a wet or soiled dressing immediately. • Change the dressing more frequently if catheter is located in femoral area or near tracheostomy. Perform tracheostomy care after catheter care. • Examine solution for cloudiness and turbidity before infusing; check the fluid container for leaks. • The catheter may be changed frequently. • Keep the system closed as much as possible.
• Notify the doctor. • Remove the catheter or assist with removal. • Administer oxygen as ordered. • Set up and assist with chest tube insertion. • Document interventions.	• Position the patient head down with a rolled towel between his scapulae to dilate and expose the internal jugular or subclavian vein as much as possible during catheter insertion. • Assess for early signs of fluid infiltration (swelling in the shoulder, neck, chest, and arm). • Make sure that the patient is immobilized and prepared for insertion. An active patient may need to be sedated or taken to the operating room.
• Clamp the catheter immediately. • Turn the patient on his left side, head down, so that air can enter the right atrium. Maintain this position for 20 to 30 minutes. • Avoid Valsalva's maneuver because a large air intake worsens the condition. • Administer oxygen. • Notify the doctor. • Document interventions.	• Purge all air from the tubing before hookup. • Teach the patient to perform Valsalva's maneuver during catheter insertion and tubing changes. • Use air-eliminating filters. • Use an infusion device with air detection capability. • Use luer-lock tubing, tape the connections, or use locking devices for all connections.
• Notify the doctor. • Possibly remove the catheter. • Possibly infuse anticoagulant doses of heparin. • Verify thrombosis with diagnostic studies. • Apply warm, wet compresses locally. • Do not use the limb on the affected side for subsequent venipuncture or blood pressure measurement. • Document interventions.	• Maintain a steady flow rate with the infusion pump, or flush the catheter at regular intervals. • Use catheters made of less thrombogenic materials or catheters coated to prevent thrombosis. • Dilute irritating solutions. • Use a 0.22-µ filter for infusions.

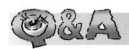

Show and tell

Identify the CV catheter insertion site in each illustration.

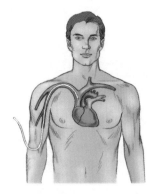

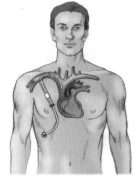

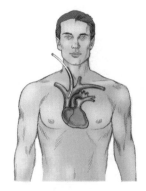

1. _____

2. _____

3. _____

Matchmaker

Match the abnormal CVP waveforms in column 2 to their descriptions in column 1.

1. Elevated a waves _____

A.

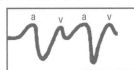

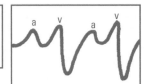

2. Absent a waves _____

B.

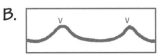

3. Elevated v waves _____

C.

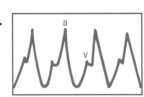

4. Elevated a and v waves _____

D.

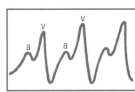

Suggested References

Alspach, J.G. (Ed.). *Core Curriculum for Critical Care Nursing*, 6th ed. Philadelphia: W.B. Saunders Co., 2006.

Arora, S., et al. "Changing Trends of Hemodynamic Monitoring in the ICU from Invasive to Non-Invasive Methods: Are We There Yet?," *International Journal of Critical Illness and Injury Science* 4(2):168–177, Apr 2014. doi: 10.4103/2229-5151.134185.

Busse, L., et al. "Hemodynamic Monitoring in the Critical Care Environment," *Advances in Chronic Kidney Disease* 20(1):21–29, Jan 2013. doi: 10.1053/j.ackd.2012.10.006.

McLaughlin, M.A. (Ed.). *Cardiovascular Care Made Incredibly Easy*, 3rd ed. Philadelphia: Lippincott Williams & Wilkins, 2014.

Carlson, K.K. (Ed.). *AACN Advanced Critical Care Nursing*. Philadelphia: Elsevier, 2009.

Chulay, M., and Burns, S.M. *AACN Essentials of Critical Care Nursing*, 3rd ed. New York: McGraw-Hill, 2014.

Diepenbrock, N. *Quick Reference to Critical Care*, 4th ed. Philadelphia: Lippincott Williams & Wilkins, 2012.

Lippincott's Nursing Procedures & Skills. Philadelphia: Lippincott Williams & Wilkins, 2009. Accessed via the online program on September 1, 2009.

Morton, P.G., and Fontaine, D.K. *Critical Care Nursing: A Holistic Approach*, 9th ed. Philadelphia: Lippincott Williams & Wilkins, 2009.

O'Grady, N.P., et al. Centers for Disease Control. 2011 Guidelines for the Prevention of Intravascular Catheter-Related Infections, 2011. Accessed from http://www.cdc.gov/hicpac/BSI/02-bsi-summary-of-recommendations-2011.html on November 14, 2014.

Scales, K., and Collie, E. "A Practical Guide to Using Pulmonary Artery Catheters," *Nursing Standard* 21(43):42–48, July 2007.

Weigand, D.L., and Carlson, K.K. *AACN Procedure Manual for Critical Care*, 6th ed. St. Louis: Elsevier Saunders, 2010.

Woods, S., et al. *Cardiac Nursing*, 6th ed. Philadelphia: Lippincott Williams & Wilkins, 2010.

Chapter 6

Pulmonary artery pressure monitoring

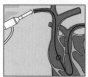
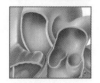
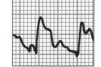

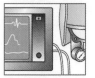

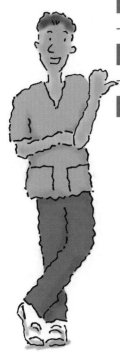

Understanding PAP and PAWP monitoring

Continuous pulmonary artery pressure (PAP) and intermittent pulmonary artery wedge pressure (PAWP) measurements provide important information about left ventricular function and preload.

The original PAP monitoring catheter, called a *Swan-Ganz catheter* or, more commonly, a *pulmonary artery (PA) catheter,* had two lumens. Current versions have up to six lumens, allowing for more hemodynamic information to be gathered.

In addition to distal and proximal lumens used to measure pressures, a PA catheter has a balloon inflation lumen that inflates the balloon for PAWP measurement and a thermistor connector lumen that enables cardiac output measurement. Some catheters also have a lumen that provides a port for a temporary pacemaker wire. Others have fiberoptic bundles that continuously measure mixed venous oxygen saturation.

A closer look at a pulmonary artery catheter

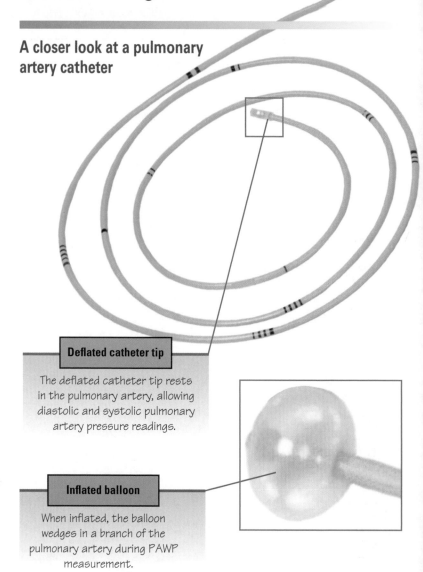

Deflated catheter tip

The deflated catheter tip rests in the pulmonary artery, allowing diastolic and systolic pulmonary artery pressure readings.

Inflated balloon

When inflated, the balloon wedges in a branch of the pulmonary artery during PAWP measurement.

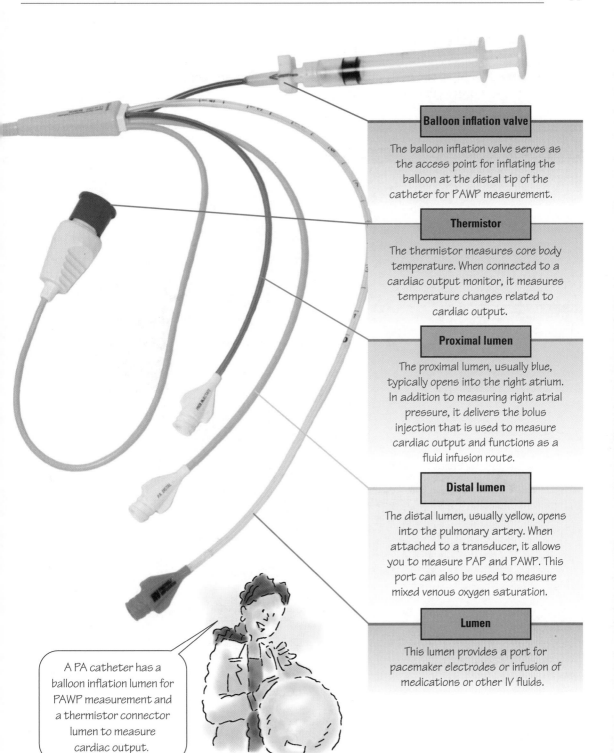

Balloon inflation valve

The balloon inflation valve serves as the access point for inflating the balloon at the distal tip of the catheter for PAWP measurement.

Thermistor

The thermistor measures core body temperature. When connected to a cardiac output monitor, it measures temperature changes related to cardiac output.

Proximal lumen

The proximal lumen, usually blue, typically opens into the right atrium. In addition to measuring right atrial pressure, it delivers the bolus injection that is used to measure cardiac output and functions as a fluid infusion route.

Distal lumen

The distal lumen, usually yellow, opens into the pulmonary artery. When attached to a transducer, it allows you to measure PAP and PAWP. This port can also be used to measure mixed venous oxygen saturation.

Lumen

This lumen provides a port for pacemaker electrodes or infusion of medications or other IV fluids.

A PA catheter has a balloon inflation lumen for PAWP measurement and a thermistor connector lumen to measure cardiac output.

A look at the whole picture...

Detecting pressure changes in the heart with a PA catheter involves the use of a fluid-filled monitoring system as described in Chapter 2. The components of this system are shown in this illustration.

Components of the PAP monitoring system

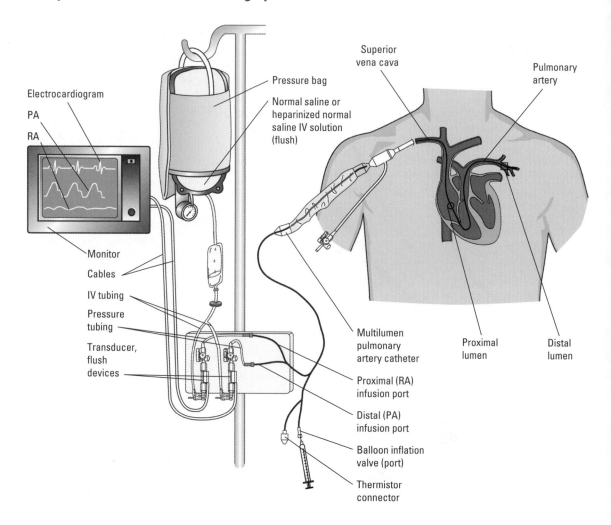

PA catheter insertion

When is PAP monitoring used?

Nearly all acutely ill patients are candidates for PAP monitoring—especially those who:

☑ are hemodynamically unstable
☑ need fluid management or continuous cardiopulmonary assessment
☑ are receiving multiple or frequently administered cardioactive drugs
☑ are in shock
☑ have experienced trauma
☑ have pulmonary, cardiac, or multisystem disease.

Cautions

Some patients require special precautions during insertion and use, including:

☑ those with left bundle-branch heart block
☑ those for whom a systemic infection would be life-threatening.

Contraindications

No specific contraindications for PAP monitoring exist. However, relative contraindications include patients with:

☑ severe coagulation disorders
☑ a prosthetic right heart valve
☑ pulmonary hypertension.

The balloon-tipped, multilumen catheter is inserted into the patient's internal jugular or subclavian vein. Fluoroscopy usually is not required during catheter insertion because the catheter is flow-directed, following venous blood flow from the right heart chambers into the pulmonary artery. Also, the pulmonary artery, right atrium, and right ventricle produce characteristic pressures and waveforms that can be observed on the monitor to help track catheter-tip location. Marks on the catheter shaft, with 10-cm graduations, assist tracking by showing how far the catheter is inserted.

When the catheter reaches the right atrium, the balloon is inflated to float the catheter through the right ventricle into the pulmonary artery. PAWP measurement is then possible through an opening at the catheter's tip. The catheter (with balloon tip deflated) rests in the pulmonary artery, allowing diastolic and systolic PAP readings. The balloon should be totally deflated except when taking a PAWP reading (prolonged wedging can cause pulmonary infarction).

Think before you act. While most patients are PAP candidates, others are not!

Fluoroscopy is not necessary with PA catheter insertion because the catheter follows venous blood flow into the pulmonary artery!

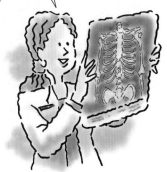

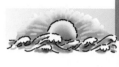

Normal pulmonary artery waveforms

After insertion into a large vein (usually the subclavian, jugular, or femoral vein), a PA catheter is advanced through the vena cava into the right atrium, through the right ventricle, and into a branch of the pulmonary artery. During insertion, the monitor shows various waveforms as the catheter advances through the heart chambers.

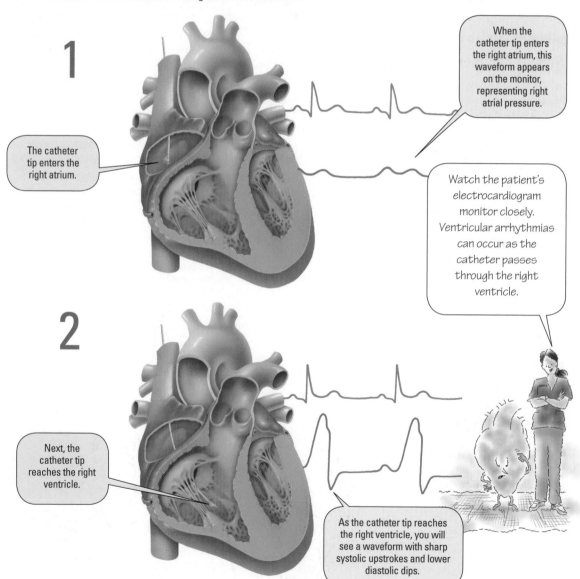

1

When the catheter tip enters the right atrium, this waveform appears on the monitor, representing right atrial pressure.

The catheter tip enters the right atrium.

Watch the patient's electrocardiogram monitor closely. Ventricular arrhythmias can occur as the catheter passes through the right ventricle.

2

Next, the catheter tip reaches the right ventricle.

As the catheter tip reaches the right ventricle, you will see a waveform with sharp systolic upstrokes and lower diastolic dips.

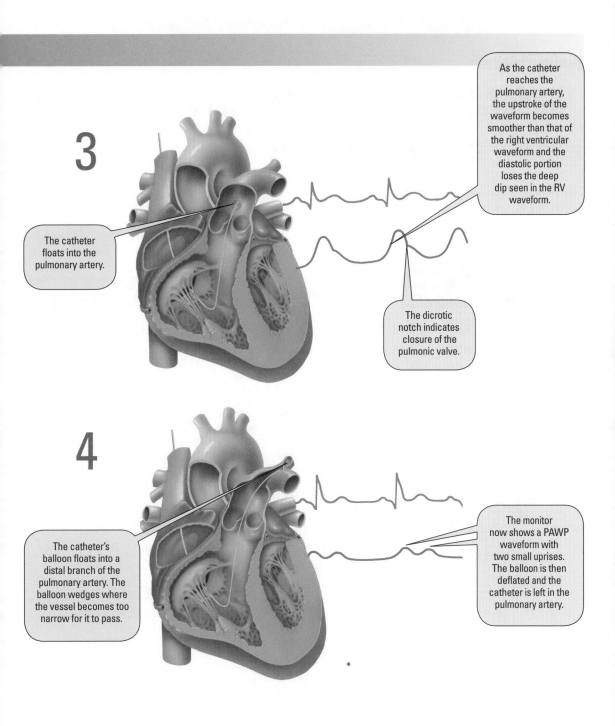

3

The catheter floats into the pulmonary artery.

As the catheter reaches the pulmonary artery, the upstroke of the waveform becomes smoother than that of the right ventricular waveform and the diastolic portion loses the deep dip seen in the RV waveform.

The dicrotic notch indicates closure of the pulmonic valve.

4

The catheter's balloon floats into a distal branch of the pulmonary artery. The balloon wedges where the vessel becomes too narrow for it to pass.

The monitor now shows a PAWP waveform with two small uprises. The balloon is then deflated and the catheter is left in the pulmonary artery.

Understanding the pulmonary artery waveform

The waveform produced by PAP monitoring is similar to the arterial pressure waveform, except that the pressures are lower (due to the lower pressures in the pulmonary arteries when compared to pressures in the systemic arteries).

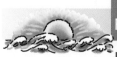

Ride the wave

PAP waveform

In this example of a normal PAP waveform, note the lower pressure scale used. This waveform would be interpreted as a PAP of 32/12 mm Hg.

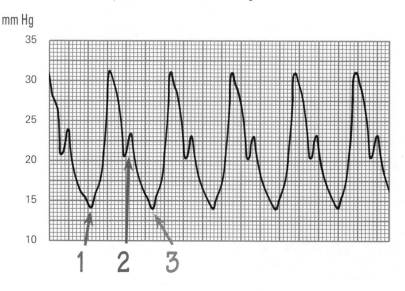

1 Systolic ejection into pulmonary artery

2 Closure of pulmonic valve (dicrotic notch)

3 End-diastole

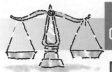

Normal PAP parameters

PAP monitoring provides information on intracardiac pressures. To understand intracardiac pressures, picture the heart and vascular system as a continuous loop with constantly changing pressure gradients that keep blood moving. PAP monitoring records the gradients within some of the heart chambers and vessels.

Pressure and description	Normal values	Causes of increased pressure	Causes of decreased pressure
Right ventricular pressure			
Typically, the doctor measures right ventricular pressure only when initially inserting a PA catheter. Right ventricular systolic pressure normally equals PA systolic pressure. Right ventricular end-diastolic pressure reflects left ventricular function.	Normal systolic pressure ranges from 20 to 30 mm Hg; normal diastolic pressure, from 0 to 5 mm Hg.	• Mitral stenosis or insufficiency • Pulmonary disease • Hypoxemia • Constrictive pericarditis • Chronic heart failure • Atrial and ventricular septal defects • Patent ductus arteriosus • Pulmonary embolus	Reduced circulating blood volume
PAP			
PA systolic pressure shows right ventricular function and pulmonary circulation pressures. PA diastolic pressure reflects left ventricular pressures, specifically left ventricular end-diastolic pressure, in a patient without significant pulmonary disease.	Systolic pressure normally ranges from 20 to 30 mm Hg; normal diastolic pressure, from 6 to 12 mm Hg. The mean pressure usually ranges from 10 to 15 mm Hg.	• Left-sided heart failure • Increased pulmonary blood flow (left or right shunting, as in atrial or ventricular septal defects) • Any condition causing increased pulmonary arteriolar resistance, such as pulmonary hypertension, volume overload, mitral stenosis, acute respiratory distress syndrome, or hypoxia	Reduced circulating blood volume
PAWP			
PAWP reflects left atrial and left ventricular pressures, unless the patient has mitral stenosis. Changes in PAWP reflect changes in left ventricular filling pressure.	The mean pressure normally ranges from 4 to 12 mm Hg.	• Left-sided heart failure • Mitral stenosis or insufficiency • Pericardial tamponade	Reduced circulating blood volume

> PAP monitoring records the gradients within some of my chambers and vessels.

A closer look at pulmonary artery pressures

After PA catheter insertion, PA systolic pressure and PA diastolic pressure are continuously monitored.

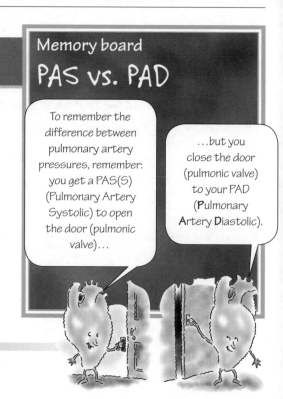

Memory board
PAS vs. PAD

To remember the difference between pulmonary artery pressures, remember: you get a PAS(S) (Pulmonary Artery Systolic) to open the door (pulmonic valve)…

…but you close the door (pulmonic valve) to your PAD (**P**ulmonary **A**rtery **D**iastolic).

Understanding pulmonary artery pressures

PA diastolic pressure
PA diastolic pressure represents the resistance of the pulmonary vascular bed as measured when the pulmonic valve is closed and the mitral valve is open. To a limited degree (under absolutely normal conditions), PA diastolic pressure also reflects left ventricular end-diastolic pressure.

PA systolic pressure
PA systolic pressure measures right ventricular systolic ejection or, simply put, the amount of pressure needed to open the pulmonic valve and eject blood into the pulmonary circulation. When the pulmonic valve is open, PA systolic pressure should be the same as right ventricular systolic pressure.

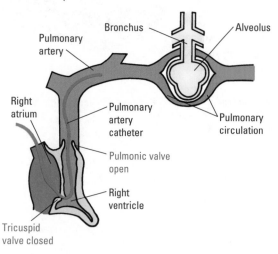

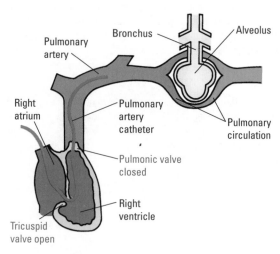

Pulmonary artery wedge pressure

PAWP reflects left atrial and left ventricular pressures. PAWP is obtained by inflating the balloon on the PA catheter tip. The balloon floats downstream with venous blood flow to a smaller, more distal branch of the pulmonary artery. Here, the catheter lodges, or *wedges,* causing occlusion in the forward flow of blood in the distal branch of the pulmonary artery. The resulting waveform resembles that of the right atrial waveform (obtained when the balloon is deflated), except that the PAWP waveform reflects back pressure from the left side of the heart.

A closer look at the wedged position

This illustration shows the positioning of the PA catheter and its inflated tip during PAWP measurement.

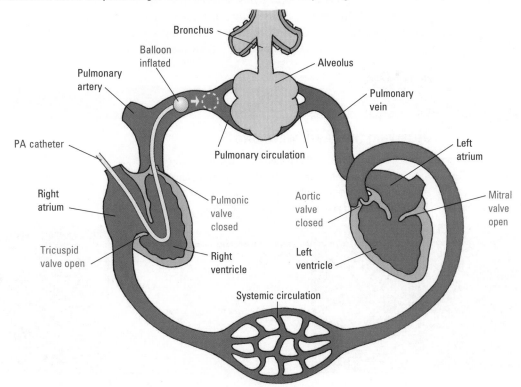

Taking a PAWP reading

By inflating the balloon and letting it float in a distal artery, you can record PAWP. Extreme caution should be used when taking a PAWP reading because of the risk of pulmonary artery rupture—a rare but life-threatening complication. Make sure that you are thoroughly familiar with intracardiac waveform interpretation and follow these steps:

1 To begin, verify that the transducer is properly leveled and zeroed. Detach the syringe from the balloon inflation hub. Draw 1.5 mL of air into the syringe, and then reattach the syringe to the hub. Watching the monitor, inject the air through the hub slowly and smoothly. When you see a wedge tracing on the monitor, immediately stop inflating the balloon. *Note:* Never inflate the balloon beyond the volume needed to obtain a wedge tracing; otherwise the pulmonary artery could rupture.

2 Take the pressure reading at end-expiration.

3 Note the amount of air needed to change the PA tracing to a wedge tracing (normally, 1.25 to 1.5 mL). If the wedge tracing appeared with injection of less than 1.25 mL, suspect that the catheter has migrated into a more distal branch and requires repositioning. If the balloon is in a more distal branch, the tracings may move up the oscilloscope, indicating that the catheter tip is recording balloon pressure rather than PAWP. This may lead to PA rupture.

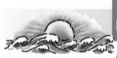

Ride the wave

Observing the PAWP waveform

Upon balloon inflation, you should see the normal PAP waveform flatten to the characteristic PAWP waveform. Balloon inflation should be halted upon observation of this waveform. Upon balloon deflation, the PAP waveform should immediately reappear. Always allow the balloon to deflate passively. Actively aspirating the air in the balloon can cause balloon rupture.

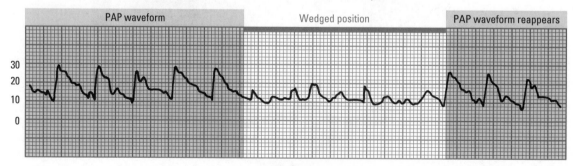

PAP waveform | Wedged position | PAP waveform reappears

Overwedging

Prolonged wedging or hyperinflation of the balloon can produce falsely elevated PAWP measurements that are useless. Prolonged wedging or hyperinflation creates occlusion of the catheter tip and distort accurate measurements by either:

- lodging the sensing tip of the catheter into the vessel wall, causing measurement of the pressure within the occluded catheter and high-pressure flush system
- causing the inflated balloon tip to become compressed by the surrounding pulmonary artery, placing pressure on the sensing tip of the catheter.

Gently now

If an overwedging waveform is noted, gently deflate the balloon tip. The PAP waveform should reappear. Then rewedge with less air, and avoid prolonged wedging.

> Overwedging is visible in a PAWP waveform that continuously rises or declines abruptly and then slowly rises again.

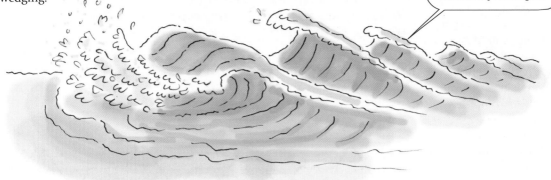

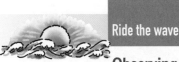 **Ride the wave**

Observing an overwedged waveform

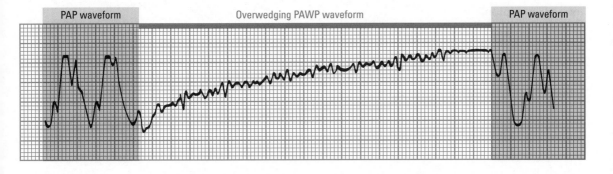

PAP waveform | Overwedging PAWP waveform | PAP waveform

Influence of intrathoracic pressure

Because the blood vessels and heart are pliable and compressible, the respiratory pressure changes that occur within the thorax may influence hemodynamic measurements. If possible, obtain PAP and PAWP values at end-expiration (when the patient completely exhales). At this time, intrathoracic pressure approaches atmospheric pressure and has the least effect on hemodynamic measurements.

If you obtain a reading during other phases of the respiratory cycle, respiratory interference may occur. For instance, during inspiration, when intrathoracic pressure drops, PAP may be false-low because the negative pressure is transmitted to the catheter. During expiration, when intrathoracic pressure rises, PAP may be false-high.

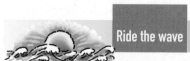

Ride the wave

Ventilatory effects on PAP and PAWP values

These waveforms illustrate how cyclical respiratory pressure changes affect PAP and PAWP measurements and highlight end-expiration points (the optimal time to obtain a reading).

Spontaneous breathing
Normal, unlabored, spontaneous respirations have a minimal effect on PAP and PAWP values, as shown below.

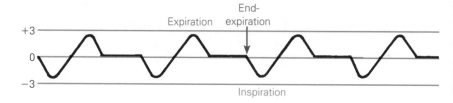

Electrocardiogram

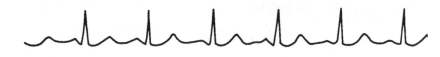

PAWP

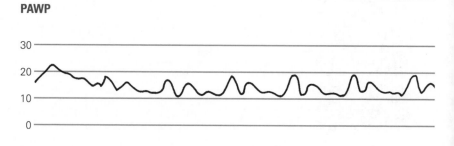

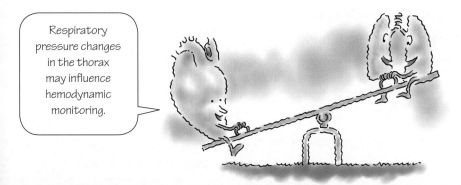

Respiratory pressure changes in the thorax may influence hemodynamic monitoring.

Mechanical ventilation

When a patient is mechanically ventilated, his PAP and PAWP waveforms will follow the intrathoracic pressure changes that occur upon delivery of ventilator breaths. Breaths delivered by a ventilator cause an increase in intrathoracic pressure during inspiration, the opposite of the pressure changes with spontaneous breaths. This diagram illustrates the effects of control mode ventilation, in which the ventilator delivers a preset tidal volume at a fixed rate, and synchronized intermittent mandatory ventilation (SIMV), in which the ventilator delivers a preset number of breaths at a specific tidal volume, but the patient may supplement these mechanical ventilations with his own breaths. The PAWP waveform baseline shows a combination of machine breaths and spontaneous breaths when the patient is ventilated using SIMV.

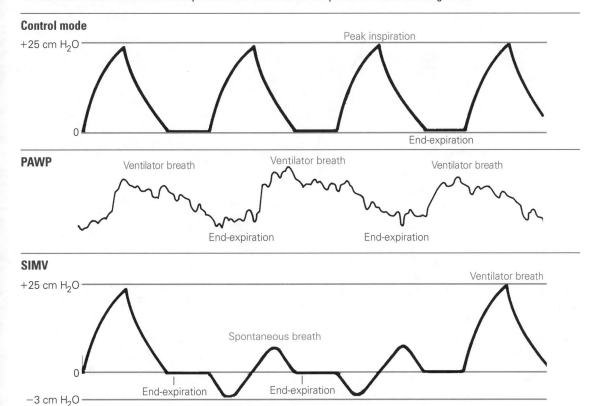

Minimizing complications of PAP monitoring

A patient who has a PA catheter in place is at risk for several complications. In addition to observing the patient's electrocardiogram, waveform pattern, and PAP values on the bedside monitor, watch for these signs and symptoms of complications. Implement appropriate care measures to resolve or prevent them.

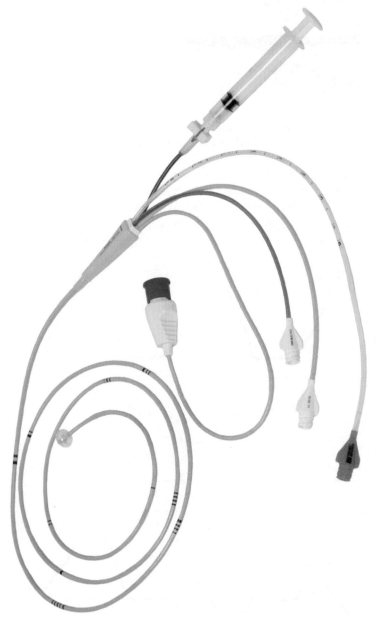

Complication and causes

Bacteremia
- Introduction of bacteria into the circulatory system

Bleedback
- Leaks in the PA catheter apparatus
- Pressure bag that is inflated below 300 mm Hg

Bleeding at the insertion site
- Inadequate application of pressure during and after catheter withdrawal

Pulmonary embolism
- Thrombus migration from the catheter into pulmonary circulation
- Clotted catheter tip from inadequate flushing

Pulmonary infarction
- Catheter migration into a wedged position in the blood vessel

Ruptured pulmonary artery
- Pulmonary hypertension
- Thrombus
- Catheter migration into a peripheral branch of the artery
- Improper inflation or prolonged wedging of the catheter's balloon

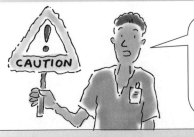

Watch for these signs and symptoms of complications from PAP monitoring.

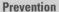

Signs and symptoms	Prevention
• Fever • Chills • Warm skin • Headache • Malaise	• Maintain strict sterile technique. • Maintain and change the monitoring setup according to facility policy.
• Blood easily seen in the pressure tubing	• Tighten all connections in the monitoring setup. • Return stopcocks to their proper position after use. • Keep the pressure bag adequately inflated.
• Prolonged oozing or frank bleeding at the insertion site after catheter withdrawal	• Maintain pressure on the site during catheter withdrawal and for at least 10 minutes afterward. • Apply a pressure dressing over the site. • At a femoral site, apply a sandbag for 1 to 2 hours. • Be sure to assess distal circulation routinely to ensure that a hematoma is not obstructing blood flow.
• Sharp, stabbing chest pain • Anxiety • Cyanosis • Dyspnea • Tachypnea • Diaphoresis	• Administer anticoagulants as ordered. • Use a continuous flush system. • If clotting of the catheter is suspected, gently aspirate blood (with clots), and then gently irrigate the line with flush solution.
• Chest pain • Hemoptysis • Fever • Pleural friction rub • Low arterial oxygen levels	• Never allow the balloon to be inflated for more than two respiratory cycles or 15 seconds. • After wedging, make sure that a clearly defined PA waveform returns on the monitor.
• Restlessness • Tachycardia • Hypotension • Hemoptysis • Dyspnea	• Slowly inflate the balloon only until the PAWP waveform appears on the monitor, and then let the balloon deflate passively. • Never overinflate the balloon. • Reposition a migrating catheter, if permitted.

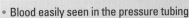

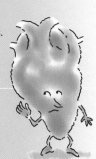

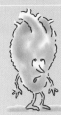

Troubleshooting the PAP monitoring system

When your patient has a PA catheter, do you know how to respond to an uncharacteristic waveform on the monitor? For example, what action should you take for an erratic waveform? How should you respond to a concurrent arrhythmia on the electrocardiogram? How can you deal with an obviously inaccurate pressure reading? Use this chart to help you recognize and resolve common problems.

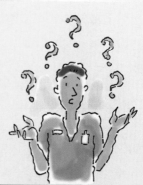

Problem	Causes	Nursing interventions
No waveform on monitor	• Transducer not open to catheter • Transducer or monitor set up improperly • Defective or cracked transducer • Clotted catheter tip • Large leak in the system; loose connections	• Check the stopcock, calibration, and scale mechanisms of the system. • Tighten all connections. • Rezero the setup. • Replace the transducer.
Overdamped waveform	• Air bubble or blood clots within the catheter or tubing • Catheter tip lodged in the vessel wall • Kinked or knotted catheter or tubing • Small leak in the system due to a loose connection	• Remove air bubbles observed in the catheter tubing and transducer. • Restore patency to a clotted catheter by gently aspirating the clot with a syringe. (*Note:* Never irrigate the line as a first step.) • Correct a lodged catheter by repositioning the patient or by having him cough and breathe deeply.
Changed waveform configuration (noisy or erratic tracings)	• Incorrectly positioned catheter • Loose connections in the setup • Faulty electrical circuitry	• Reposition the patient. • Assist with chest X-ray to verify catheter location. • Check and tighten connections in the catheter and transducer apparatus.
Ventricular irritability (PVCs or V Tach)	• Irritation of the ventricular endocardium or heart valves by the catheter	• Notify the provider. (*Note:* The provider may prevent this problem during insertion by keeping the balloon inflated when advancing the catheter through the heart.) • Administer antiarrhythmic drugs as ordered. • Verify that the pressure waveform is not the RV waveform.
Right ventricular waveform	• Migration of the PA catheter into the right ventricle	• Notify the provider immediately. The catheter may need to be repositioned.

Problem	Causes	Nursing interventions
Catheter fling	• Excessive catheter movement that may result from an arrhythmia, excessive respiratory effort, hyperdynamic circulation, excessive catheter length in the right ventricle, or location of the catheter tip near the pulmonic valve	• Notify the provider for catheter repositioning.
Falsely increased or decreased pressure readings	• System not properly leveled or zeroed • Patient's body or bed repositioned without releveling or rezeroing the system	• Reposition the transducer level with the phlebostatic axis. • Rezero the monitor.
Continuous PAWP waveform	• Catheter migration • Balloon still inflated	• Verify that the balloon is deflated. • Reposition the patient or have him cough and breathe deeply. • Keep the balloon inflated for no longer than two respiratory cycles or 15 seconds.
Missing PAWP waveform	• Malpositioned catheter • Insufficient air in the balloon tip • Ruptured balloon	• Reposition the patient. (Do not aspirate the balloon.) • Reinflate the balloon adequately. (Remove the syringe from the balloon lumen, wait for the balloon to deflate passively, and then instill the correct volume of air.) • Assess the balloon's competence. (Note resistance during inflation, feel how the syringe's plunger springs back after the balloon inflates, and check for blood leaking from the balloon lumen.) • If the balloon has ruptured, turn the patient onto his left side, tape the balloon-inflation port, and notify the doctor.

Nursing Responsibilities in PAP monitoring

Maintain the monitoring system	• Keep the pressure on the flush bag > 300 mm Hg. • Ensure that there is fluid in the flush bag. It will be depleted over time. • Keep the balloon tip deflated unless wedging. • Never infuse medications or fluids through the PA distal lumen. • Continuously monitor the PA waveform.
Maintain accuracy of readings	• Prime the tubing and transducer carefully to avoid or remove air bubbles in the system. • Ensure the correct pressure scales on the monitor are used. • Level and zero the transducers every shift and with position changes. • Obtain pressures at end-expiration. • Inflate the balloon tip only long enough to get the wedge reading. • Use only the syringe provided with the PA catheter for wedge readings. • Note the level of catheter insertion each shift.
Prevent infection	• Ensure aseptic technique with maximal barrier precautions during PA catheter insertion. • Follow your facility's policies and procedures for accessing the PA catheter lumens. • Observe the insertion site for redness, swelling, or other signs of infection. • Monitor patient temperature while the catheter is in place.
Patient and family education	• Inform them of the purpose of the PA catheter and the rationale for using. • Let family members know how they can safely interact with the patient to avoid accidental dislodgement of the PA catheter.

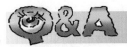

Matchmaker

Match the PAP monitoring problem to the possible cause.

1. Overdamped waveform _____

2. Right ventricular waveform _____

3. Falsely increased or decreased
   pressure readings _____

4. Missing PAWP waveform _____

A. Insufficient air in the balloon tip

B. Migration of the PA catheter into the right ventricle

C. Catheter tip lodged in the vessel wall

D. Patient's body or bed repositioned without
   releveling or rezeroing the system

Show and tell

Identify the waveforms in each illustration.

1. _____

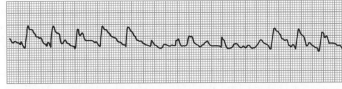

2. _____

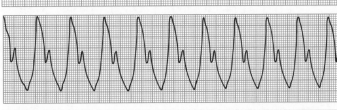

3. _____

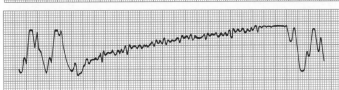

What do you know?

1. Your patient had a PA catheter placed earlier today. What would
   you do if you saw the following waveform on the monitor?

_____

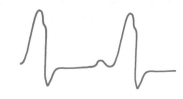

2. What is the PAWP pressure on this spontaneously breathing patient?

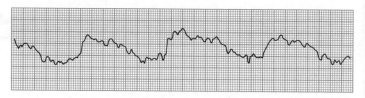

_____

3. Which hemodynamic parameter can be used instead of the PAWP to assess left ventricular function?

_____

Answers: Matchmaker: 1. C, 2. B, 3. D, 4. A. Show and tell: 1. Normal PAWP waveform, 2. Normal PAP waveform, 3. Overwedged waveform. What do you know? 1. Notify the physician to reposition the PA catheter. The tip has migrated to the right ventricle. 2. I can determine the answer when the waveform is available. 3. Pulmonary artery diastolic pressure (PAD).

Suggested References

Alspach, J.G. (Ed.). *Core Curriculum for Critical Care Nursing*, 6th ed. Philadelphia: W.B. Saunders Co., 2006.

Arora, S., et al. "Changing Trends of Hemodynamic Monitoring in the ICU- from Invasive to Non-invasive Methods: Are We There Yet?" *International Journal of Critical Illness and Injury Science*; 4(2):168–177, April 2014. doi:10.4103/2229-5151.134185.

Busse, L., et al. "Hemodynamic Monitoring in the Critical Care Environment," *Advances in Chronic Kidney Disease*; 20(1):21–29, January 2013. doi:10.1053/j.ackd.2012.10.006.

Carlson, K.K. (Ed.). *AACN Advanced Critical Care Nursing*. Philadelphia: Elsevier, 2009.

Centers for Disease Control. 2011 Guidelines for the Prevention of Intravascular Catheter-Related Infections. http://www.cdc.gov/hicpac/BSI/02-bsi-summary-of-recommendations-2011.html. Accessed November 14, 2014.

Chulay, M., and Burns, S.M. *AACN Essentials of Critical Care Nursing*, 3rd ed. New York: McGraw-Hill, 2014.

Diepenbrock, N. *Quick Reference to Critical Care*, 4th ed. Philadelphia: Lippincott Williams & Wilkins, 2012.

Lippincott's Nursing Procedures & Skills. Philadelphia: Lippincott Williams & Wilkins, 2009. Accessed via the online program on September 1, 2009.

McLaughlin, M.A. (Ed.). *Cardiovascular Care Made Incredibly Easy*, 3rd ed. Philadelphia: Lippincott Williams & Wilkins, 2014.

Morton, P.G., and Fontaine, D.K. *Critical Care Nursing: A Holistic Approach*, 9th ed. Philadelphia: Lippincott Williams & Wilkins, 2009.

Scales, K., and Collie, E. "A Practical Guide to Using Pulmonary Artery Catheters," *Nursing Standard* 21(43):42–48, July 2007.

Weigand, D.L., and Carlson, K.K. *AACN Procedure Manual for Critical Care*, 6th ed. St. Louis: Elsevier Saunders, 2010.

Woods, S., et al. *Cardiac Nursing*, 6th ed. Philadelphia: Lippincott Williams & Wilkins, 2010.

Chapter 7

Cardiac output monitoring

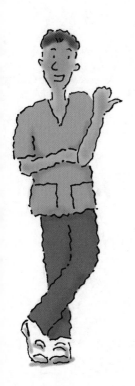
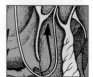
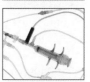

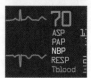

Understanding cardiac output monitoring

Measuring cardiac output

Measuring cardiac output (CO)—the amount of blood ejected by the heart over 1 minute—helps evaluate cardiac function. Cardiac output is a function of heart rate multipled by stroke volume, and the three major components of stroke volume are preload, afterload, and contractility. The most widely used method for monitoring CO is the thermodilution technique, either bolus or continuous. Performed at the bedside, the thermodilution technique is the most practical method of evaluating the cardiac status of critically ill patients and those suspected of having cardiac disease, and is the method focused on in this chapter. The Fick method can also be used to measure or estimate cardiac output.

Methods of measuring cardiac output

Fick method

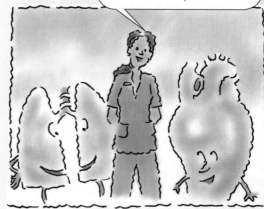

The Fick method is useful in detecting or estimating cardiac output levels. Cardiac output is calculated based on arterial and venous oxygen levels and oxygen consumption.

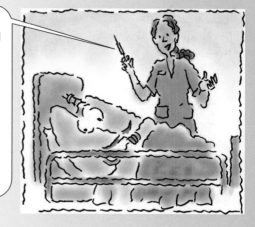

First, arterial and venous blood samples are obtained and analyzed for oxygen content. Arterial blood can be obtained from any convenient arterial source, or if no invasive specimen can be obtained, a reliable arterial pulse oximetry value can be substituted. Venous blood samples should be obtained from either the pulmonary artery or the right atrium.

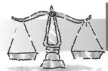

On the level

What causes changes in cardiac output?

Normally, CO ranges from 4 to 8 L/min. Values below this range may result from:
- decreased myocardial contractility caused by myocardial damage, drug effects, acidosis, or hypoxia
- decreased left ventricular filling pressure (reduced preload) resulting from hypovolemia
- increased systemic vascular resistance (increased afterload) related to arteriosclerosis or hypertension
- decreased ventricular flow related to valvular heart disease.
- High CO can occur with some arteriovenous shunts and from decreased vascular resistance (as in septic shock).

In some cases, an unusually high CO can be normal—for example, in well-conditioned athletes.

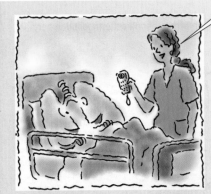

Then, a spirometer measures oxygen consumption, which is the amount of oxygen used by the tissues of the body each minute. In some cases, oxygen consumption is estimated at 125 mL/min at rest.

$$CO \ (L/min) = \frac{oxygen \ consumption \ (mL/min)}{arterial \ oxygen \ content \ (mL/min) - venous \ oxygen \ content \ (mL/min)}$$

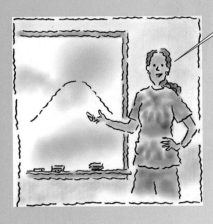

To calculate CO, these values are entered into a formula or a computer performs the computation.

Thermodilution methods

Bedside CO measurements are obtained by an intermittent bolus method or a continuous CO (CCO) method.

A closer look at the intermittent bolus thermodilution method

To measure CO using the intermittent bolus thermodilution method, a quantity of solution at least 10 degrees cooler than the patient's blood is injected into the right atrium through the proximal injectate (blue) or central venous port on a PA catheter. This indicator solution mixes with the blood as it travels through the right ventricle into the pulmonary artery, and a thermistor on the catheter registers the change in temperature of the flowing blood. A computer then plots the temperature change over time as a curve and calculates flow based on the area under the curve.

This illustration shows the path of the injectate solution through the heart during intermittent bolus thermodilution cardiac output monitoring.

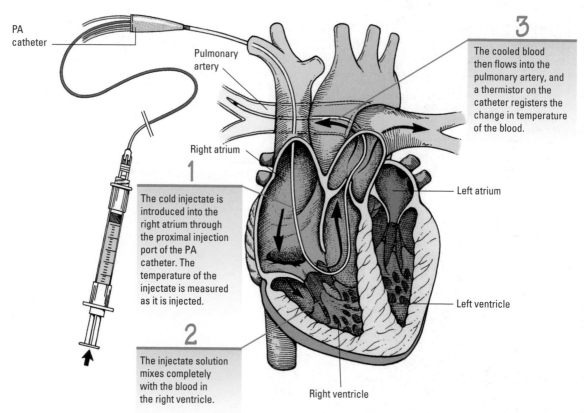

PA catheter

Pulmonary artery

Right atrium

1
The cold injectate is introduced into the right atrium through the proximal injection port of the PA catheter. The temperature of the injectate is measured as it is injected.

2
The injectate solution mixes completely with the blood in the right ventricle.

3
The cooled blood then flows into the pulmonary artery, and a thermistor on the catheter registers the change in temperature of the blood.

Left atrium

Left ventricle

Right ventricle

Intermittent bolus thermodilution setup

Equipment and supplies used for this thermodilution method include a thermodilution PA catheter in position, an output computer and cables (or a module for the bedside cardiac monitor), a closed or open injectate delivery system, a 10-mL syringe, a 500-mL bag of injectate solution (typically 0.9% sodium chloride), and crushed ice and water or cooling unit (if iced injectant is to be used).

PA catheter prepared for CO monitoring

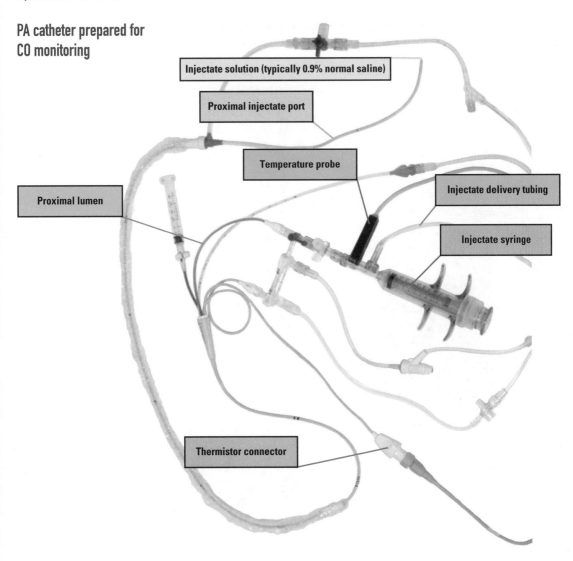

- Injectate solution (typically 0.9% normal saline)
- Proximal injectate port
- Temperature probe
- Injectate delivery tubing
- Injectate syringe
- Proximal lumen
- Thermistor connector

A closer look at the continuous cardiac output method

Measuring CO using a continuous cardiac output (CCO) system requires a modified pulmonary artery catheter and CO computer. Rather than using a cooler-than-blood injectant as the input signal, the CCO system relies on a thermal filament on the catheter's outer surface. The thermal filament creates an input signal by emitting pulses of low heat energy, warming blood as it flows by; a thermistor then measures the temperature downstream. A computer algorithm identifies when the pulmonary artery temperature change matches the temperature of the input signal and produces a thermodilution washout curve and the CO value.

The monitor measures CO about every 30 to 60 seconds and displays a continuously updated CO value, averaged from the previous 3 to 6 minutes of data collected.

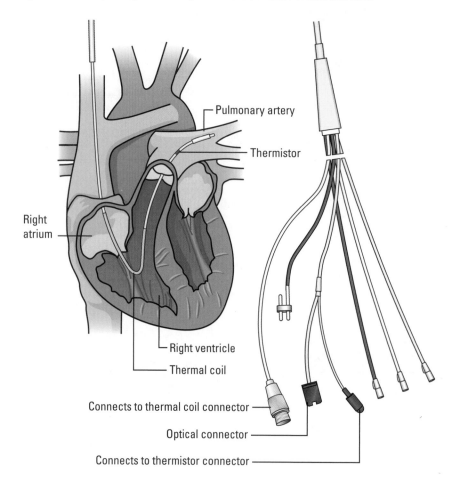

Pulmonary artery

Thermistor

Right atrium

Right ventricle

Thermal coil

Connects to thermal coil connector

Optical connector

Connects to thermistor connector

Measuring an intermittent bolus cardiac output

Room-temperature injectate with a closed delivery system

Position the patient in the supine position with head of bed between 0 to 20 degrees.

• Connect the primed system to the stopcock of the proximal injectate lumen of the PA catheter. Consider presence of any infusions also infusing through the proximal injectate lumen. Relocate medicated infusions to alternative infusion sites.

• Connect the temperature probe from the CO computer to the closed injectate system's flow-through housing device.

• Connect the CO computer cable to the thermistor connector on the PA catheter and verify the blood temperature reading.

• Turn on the CO computer and enter the correct computation constant as provided by the catheter's manufacturer. The constant is determined by the volume and temperature of the injectate as well as the size and type of catheter. Ensure that the computation constant is specific to the volume and temperature of the injectate that is being used. (An example of a computation constant table would be good here . . . to highlight what one looks like).

• Verify that the injectate temperature is at least 10 degrees cooler than the patient's blood temperature.

• Verify the presence of central venous and pulmonary artery waveforms on the cardiac monitor to verify proper position of the pulmonary artery catheter.

• Withdraw exactly 10 ml (or alternate volume) of injectate.

• Turn the stopcock at the catheter injectate hub to open a fluid path between the injectate lumen of the PA catheter and the syringe.

• Press the START button on the CO computer or wait for the INJECT message to display. Observe the patient's respiratory pattern. Then inject the solution at end-expiration smoothly within 4 seconds, making sure that it does not leak at the connectors.

• If available, analyze the contour of the thermodilution washout curve on a strip chart recorder for a rapid upstroke and a gradual, smooth return to baseline.

• Wait 1 to 2 minutes between injections or until the CO computer displays that it is ready for a new injection. Repeat the procedure until three values are 10% to 15% of the median value. Compute the average and record the patient's CO.

• Return the stopcock to its original position and make sure that the injectate delivery system is clamped.

• Verify the presence of central venous and pulmonary artery waveforms on the cardiac monitor.

Repeat bolus cardiac output measurements every 4 hours, as ordered by provider, or clinically indicated.

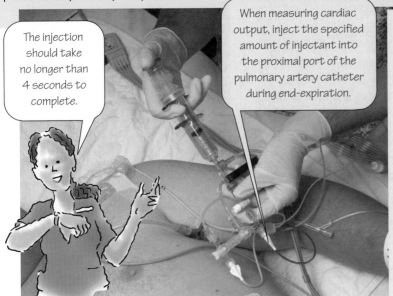

The injection should take no longer than 4 seconds to complete.

When measuring cardiac output, inject the specified amount of injectant into the proximal port of the pulmonary artery catheter during end-expiration.

Injectate considerations

Iced or room-temperature injectate may be used. The choice should be based on facility policy as well as the patient's status. The accuracy of the bolus thermodilution technique depends on the computer being able to differentiate the temperature change caused by the injectate in the pulmonary artery. Because iced injectate is colder than room-temperature injectate, it provides a stronger signal to be detected.

Iced injectate with a closed delivery system

• Place the coiled segment of the tubing into the Styrofoam container and add crushed ice and water to cover the entire coil or use a cooling unit supplied by the manufacturer.
• Let the solution cool for 15 to 20 minutes.
• Proceed as for the room-temperature injectate with a closed delivery system.

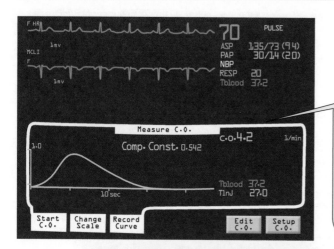

Check the thermodilution curve on the patient's monitor to make sure that the injection was properly performed. You should see a smooth, sharp rise in the curve. Repeat the injection procedure at least 3 times to obtain a mean cardiac output value.

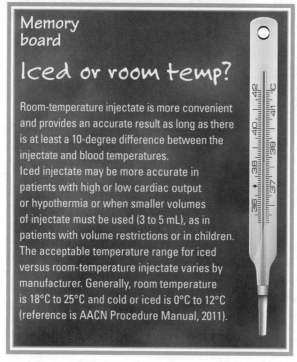

Memory board

Iced or room temp?

Room-temperature injectate is more convenient and provides an accurate result as long as there is at least a 10-degree difference between the injectate and blood temperatures.
Iced injectate may be more accurate in patients with high or low cardiac output or hypothermia or when smaller volumes of injectate must be used (3 to 5 mL), as in patients with volume restrictions or in children. The acceptable temperature range for iced versus room-temperature injectate varies by manufacturer. Generally, room temperature is 18°C to 25°C and cold or iced is 0°C to 12°C (reference is AACN Procedure Manual, 2011).

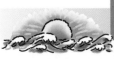

Analyzing thermodilution curves

The thermodilution curve provides valuable information about CO, injection technique, and equipment problems. When studying the curve, keep in mind that the area under the curve is inversely proportionate to CO: The smaller the area under the curve, the higher the CO; the larger the area under the curve, the lower the CO.

Besides providing a record of CO, the curve may indicate problems related to technique, such as erratic or slow injectate instillations, or other problems, such as respiratory variations or electrical interference. The curves shown here correspond to those typically seen in clinical practice.

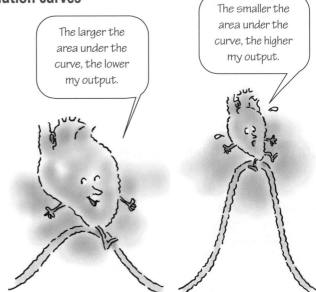

Normal thermodilution curve

With an accurate monitoring system and a patient who has adequate CO, the thermodilution curve begins with a smooth, rapid upstroke and rounded peak, and is followed by a smooth, gradual downslope. The curve shown below indicates that the injectate instillation time was within the recommended 4 seconds and that the temperature curve returned to baseline blood temperature.

The height of the curve will vary, depending on whether you use a room-temperature or an iced injectate. Room-temperature injectate produces an upstroke of lower amplitude.

Low CO curve

A thermodilution curve representing low CO shows a rapid, smooth upstroke (from proper injection technique). However, because the heart is ejecting blood less efficiently from the ventricles, the injectate warms slowly and takes longer to be ejected from the ventricle. Consequently, the curve takes longer to return to baseline. This slow return produces a larger area under the curve, corresponding to low CO.

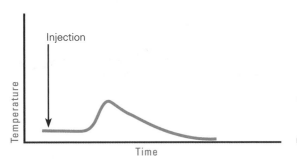

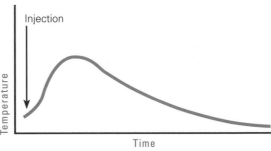

High CO curve

Again, the curve has a rapid, smooth upstroke from proper injection technique. But because the ventricles are ejecting blood too forcefully, the injectate moves through the heart quickly and the curve returns to baseline more rapidly. The smaller area under the curve suggests higher CO.

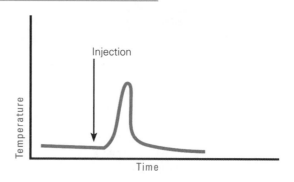

Curve reflecting poor technique

This curve results from an uneven and too slow (taking more than 4 seconds) administration of injectate. The uneven and slower-than-normal upstroke and the larger area under the curve erroneously indicate low CO. A kinked catheter, unsteady hands during the injection, or improper placement of the injectate lumen in the introducer sheath may also cause this type of curve.

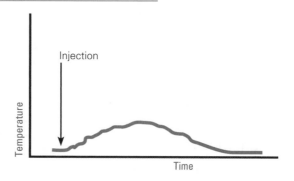

Curve associated with respiratory variations

To obtain a reliable CO measurement, you need a steady baseline pulmonary artery blood temperature. If the patient has rapid or labored respirations or if he is receiving mechanical ventilation, the thermodilution curve may reflect inaccurate CO values. The curve shown below from a patient receiving mechanical ventilation reflects fluctuating pulmonary artery blood temperatures. The thermistor interprets the unsteady temperature as a return to baseline. The result is a curve erroneously showing a high CO (small area under the curve). (*Note:* In some cases, the equipment senses no return to baseline at all and produces a sinelike curve recorded by the computer as 0.00.)

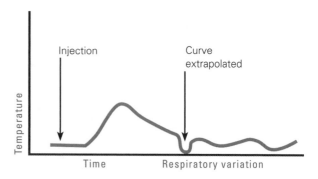

Measuring cardiac function

Once cardiac output measurement is completed, other hemodynamics parameters can be calculated to complete the hemodynamic profile. Values needed to complete the hemodynamic profile include the patient's body surface area (BSA), mean arterial pressure (MAP), central venous (or right atrial) pressure, mean pulmonary artery pressure (MPAP), and pulmonary artery wedge pressure (PAWP). Calculate the cardiac index, stroke volume (SV), stroke volume index (SVI), systemic vascular resistance (SVR), or pulmonary vascular resistance (PVR) using the prescribed formulas. For continuity, the same values for CO, heart rate (HR), and SV will be used throughout the equations. Keep in mind that most monitoring systems compute these values automatically.

Body surface area nomogram

To use the nomogram, locate the patient's height in the left column of the nomogram and weight in the right column and use a ruler to draw a straight line connecting the two points. The point where the line intersects the surface area column indicates the patient's BSA in square meters.

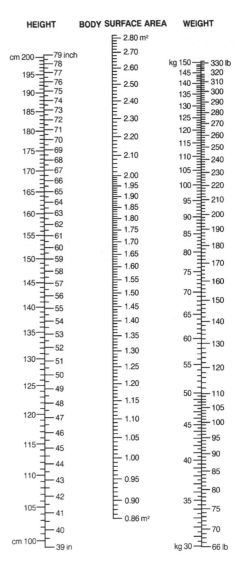

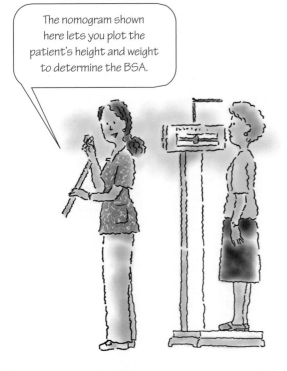

The nomogram shown here lets you plot the patient's height and weight to determine the BSA.

Calculating the cardiac index (CI)

Because it takes into account the patient's size, the CI is a more accurate indicator of CO. To calculate the CI, divide the CO value by the patient's BSA. Normally, the CI ranges from 2.5 to 4 L/min/m² (of BSA). For example, a patient's cardiac output is 5.5 L/min and BSA is 1.64. Cardiac index would be 5.5/1.64 or 3.36 L/min/m².

1 Stroke volume

To determine SV—the volume of blood pumped by the ventricle in one contraction—multiply the CO by 1,000 and divide by the HR. Normal SV ranges between 60 and 100 mL/beat.

$$SV = \frac{CO \times 1,000}{HR}$$

Example
Here, the patient's CO is 5.5 L/min and his HR is 80 beats/min.

$$SV = \frac{5.5 \times 1,000}{80}$$

$$SV = \frac{5,500}{80}$$

$$SV = 68.75 \text{ mL/beat}$$

2 Stroke volume index (SVI)

To assess whether the patient's SV is adequate for his body size, compute the SVI. Do so by dividing the SV by the patient's body surface area (BSA) or dividing his cardiac index (CI) $\times$ 1,000 by his HR. Normally, the SVI ranges between 35 and 75 mL/beat/m^2 of BSA.

$$SVI = \frac{SV}{BSA}$$

or

$$SVI = \frac{CI}{HR} \times 1,000$$

Example
As we determined in the example above, the patient's SV is 68.75 mL/beat. His BSA is 1.64 m^2 and his CI is 3.35 L/min/m^2.

$$SV = \frac{68.75}{1.64}$$

$$SVI = 42 \text{ mL/beat/m}^2$$

or

$$SV = \frac{3.35}{80} \times 1,000$$

$$SVI = 42 \text{ mL/beat/m}^2$$

3 Systemic vascular resistance

To assess SVR—the degree of left ventricular resistance known as *afterload*—deduct the central venous pressure (CVP) from the MAP. Divide this value by the CO value. Then multiply by a rounded conversion factor of 80 to compute the value into units of force (dynes/sec/cm^{25}). Normal SVR ranges from 800 to 1,500 dynes/sec/cm^{25}.

$$SVR = \frac{MAP - CVP}{CO} \times 80$$

Example
Here the patient's MAP is 93 and his CVP is 6; CO remains 5.5. Note that 80 is the conversion factor.

$$SVR = \frac{93 - 6}{5.5} \times 80$$

$$SVR = \frac{6,960}{5.5}$$

$$SVR = 1,265 \ dynes/sec/cm^{-5}$$

4 Pulmonary vascular resistance

To measure PVR—or right ventricular afterload—deduct the PAWP from the MPAP. Then divide the product by the CO value. To compute the value into units of force (dynes/sec/cm^{25}), multiply the result by 80. Normal PVR values range from 155 to 250 dynes/sec/cm^{25}.

$$PVR = \frac{MPAP - PAWP}{CO} \times 80$$

Example
Here, the patient's MPAP is 20 and his PAWP is 5; his CO remains 5.5. Again, the conversion factor is 80.

$$PVR = \frac{20 - 5}{5.5} \times 80$$

$$PVR = \frac{1,200}{5.5}$$

$$PVR = 218 \ dynes/sec/cm^{-5}$$

Nursing Responsibilities

- Maintain pulmonary artery catheter per institutional guidelines.
- Monitor right atrium and pulmonary artery waveforms to verify proper catheter position.
- Measure and document cardiac output and other hemodynamic parameters as prescribed or indicated.
- Include the fluid volume used for bolus cardiac output measurement in the patient's intake and output.
- Change the system components (injectate tubing, solution, etc.) with the hemodynamic monitoring system (every 96 hours).
- Correlate changes in hemodynamic measurements with changes in patient condition and/or medication administration.

Problem	Causes	Nursing interventions
CO values lower than expected	Injectate volume greater than indicated for computation constant	• Be sure to instill only the injectate volume that is appropriate for the computation constant (CC).
	Erroneous computation constant (set too low)	• Before injection, verify that the CC setting and the injectate volume are compatible.
	Injectate lumen exiting in right ventricle	• Confirm proper placement of the injectate lumen by observing the monitor for right atrial waveforms.
CO values higher than expected	Injectate volume smaller than indicated for computation constant	• Before injection, verify that the injectate volume is correct for the determined CC. • Look for and expel air bubbles from the injectate syringe.
	Erroneous computation constant (set too high)	• Before injection, verify that the CC setting and the injectate volume are compatible.
	Catheter tip too far into pulmonary artery	• Check catheter placement by obtaining a PAWP tracing. If the catheter is placed correctly, 1.25 to 1.5 mL of air will be necessary to obtain a PAWP tracing. • Assist the doctor to reposition the catheter if necessary.
CO values deviating at least 10% from the mean (no pattern)	Arrhythmias, such as premature ventricular contractions and atrial fibrillation	• Observe the electrocardiogram monitor while monitoring CO, and try to instill injectate during a period without arrhythmias. • Increase the number of serial injections to five or six, and average the values. • If the arrhythmias continue, notify the doctor.
	Catheter fling (turbulent, erratic waveform resulting from turbulence of blood circulating around intrusive catheter)	• Observe the waveforms, and assist the doctor in repositioning the catheter if necessary. • If catheter fling does not decrease spontaneously after the catheter is inserted or repositioned, increase the number of serial CO determinations.

Problem	Causes	Nursing interventions
	Varying pulmonary artery baseline temperature (which causes drift during respiration)	• Obtain CO values when respirations are steadier and less labored. • Minimize temperature variations by administering injectate during the same phase of the respiratory cycle each time you measure CO. • Increase the number of serial injections.
	Variations in venous return (for example, from rapid bolus administration of fluids or from the patient shivering, or coughing.)	• Avoid giving bolus injections of drugs or fluids just before measuring CO. • If shivering accompanies a fever, notify the doctor. • Avoid measuring CO until coughing and restlessness subside.
	Inadequate signal-to-noise ratio	• To strengthen the signal, increase the injectate volume or lower the injectate temperature (for example, by using iced injectate for patients with hypothermia).
	Poor injection technique	• Observe the upstroke on the thermodilution curve to detect an error in injection technique. • Use two hands to deliver a bolus injection quickly and evenly in less than 4 seconds.

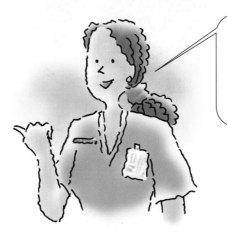

Cardiac output that falls below or above the mean can signal trouble. Follow these troubleshooting steps to avoid inaccurate measurements.

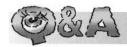

Color my world

Use a red pen or pencil to trace the path of injectate through the heart illustrated here.

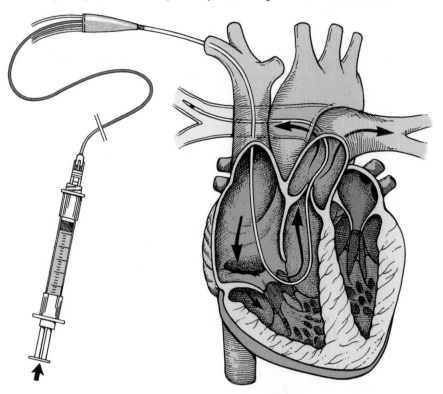

1. The two most common methods of cardiac output measurement are:
    A. _____
    B. _____

2. Which of the following statements is a technique used when measuring bolus thermodilution cardiac output?
    A. Inject volume over 15 seconds at end-inspiration.
    B. Ensure correct computation constant is utilized.
    C. Inject volume into the pulmonary artery port.
    D. Ensure temperature difference of less than 10 degrees.

Matchmaker

Match the following parameters with their descriptions.

1. stroke volume _____

2. systemic vascular resistance _____

3. pulmonary vascular resistance _____

4. cardiac index _____

A. Reflects left ventricular afterload

B. Cardiac output reflective of patients height and weight

C. Volume of blood pumped by the ventricle in one contraction

D. Reflects right ventricular afterload

Answers: Color my world: The cold injectate is introduced into the right atrium through the proximal injection port. Then it flows into the right ventricle where it mixes completely with the blood. Lastly, it flows into the pulmonary artery. Questions: 1. A. Fick equation B. Thermodilution, 2. B. Matchmaker: 1. C, 2. A, 3. D, 4. B.

Suggested References

Alspach, J.G. (Ed.). *Core Curriculum for Critical Care Nursing*, 6th ed. Philadelphia: W.B. Saunders Co., 2006.

Arora, S., et al. "Changing Trends of Hemodynamic Monitoring in the ICU- from Invasive to Non-invasive Methods: Are We There Yet?" *International Journal of Critical Illness and Injury Science*; 4(2):168–177, April 2014. doi:10.4103/2229-5151.134185.

Busse, L., et al. "Hemodynamic Monitoring in the Critical Care Environment," *Advances in Chronic Kidney Disease*; 20(1):21–29, January 2013. doi:10.1053/j.ackd.2012.10.006.

McLaughlin, M.A. (Ed.). *Cardiovascular Care Made Incredibly Easy*, 3rd ed. Philadelphia: Lippincott Williams & Wilkins, 2014.

Carlson, K.K. (Ed.). *AACN Advanced Critical Care Nursing*. Philadelphia: Elsevier, 2009.

Centers for Disease Control. 2011 Guidelines for the Prevention of Intravascular Catheter-Related Infections. http://www.cdc.gov/hicpac/BSI/02-bsi-summary-of-recommendations-2011.html. Accessed November 14, 2014.

Chulay, M., and Burns, S.M. *AACN Essentials of Critical Care Nursing*, 3rd ed. New York: McGraw-Hill, 2014.

Diepenbrock, N. *Quick Reference to Critical Care*, 4th ed. Philadelphia: Lippincott Williams & Wilkins, 2012.

Lippincott's Nursing Procedures & Skills. Philadelphia: Lippincott Williams & Wilkins, 2009. Accessed via the online program on September 1, 2009.

Morton, P.G., and Fontaine, D.K. *Critical Care Nursing: A Holistic Approach*, 9th ed. Philadelphia: Lippincott Williams & Wilkins, 2009.

Scales, K., and Collie, E. "A Practical Guide to Using Pulmonary Artery Catheters," *Nursing Standard* 21(43):42–48, July 2007.

Weigand, D.L., and Carlson, K.K. *AACN Procedure Manual for Critical Care*, 6th ed. St. Louis: Elsevier Saunders, 2010.

Woods, S., et al. *Cardiac Nursing*, 6th ed. Philadelphia: Lippincott Williams & Wilkins, 2010.

Chapter 8

Tissue oxygenation monitoring

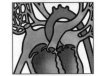

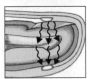

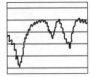

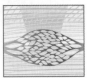

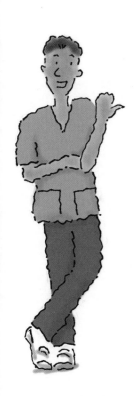

Understanding oxygen supply and tissue demand

Most oxygen (O_2) collected in the lungs binds with hemoglobin (Hb) to form oxyhemoglobin. However, a small portion of it dissolves in the plasma. The portion of oxygen that dissolves in the plasma can be measured as the partial pressure of arterial oxygen in the blood (PaO_2).

After oxygen binds to Hb, red blood cells (RBCs) carry it by way of the circulatory system to tissues throughout the body. Internal respiration occurs by cellular diffusion when RBCs release oxygen and absorb the carbon dioxide (CO_2) produced by cellular metabolism. The RBCs then transport the carbon dioxide back to the lungs for removal during expiration.

> Most of the oxygen I collect binds with hemoglobin to form oxyhemoglobin.

Oxygen and carbon dioxide transport

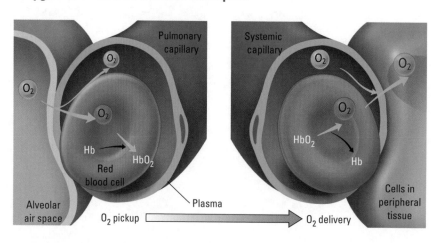

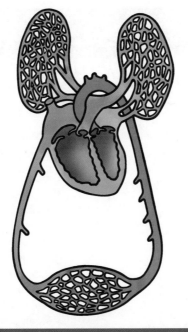

Venous oxygen reserve

Venous oxygen reserve (Rvo_2) is the amount of oxygen left over (not used by body tissues) that returns to the heart in venous blood. Rvo_2 depends on two factors:
• arterial oxygen delivery (Dao_2)
• oxygen consumption.
Normal Rvo_2 ranges from 700 to 800 mL O_2/min, or 450 mL O_2/min/m² based on body surface area (BSA).

Arterial oxygen delivery

The amount of oxygen transported to the tissues, Dao_2, depends on two factors:
• arterial oxygen content as reflected from the total amount of oxygen in the blood that is available at the cellular level.
• cardiac output defined as the amount of blood pumped out of the heart per minute.
Normal Dao_2 ranges from 900 to 1,000 mL O_2/min, or 600 mL O_2/min/m² based on BSA.

Oxygen consumption

The amount of oxygen used by the tissues in the body is called *oxygen consumption*. Oxygen consumption is determined by three factors:
• oxygen demand
• oxygen delivery
• oxygen transport
In relative terms, the cells' requirement for oxygen requires timely, efficient delivery of adequate supplies of oxygen. Normal oxygen consumption ranges from 200 to 240 mL O_2/min, or 150 mL O_2/min/m² based on BSA.

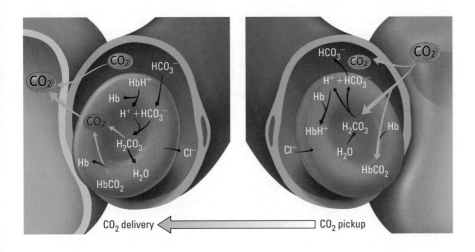

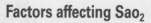

A closer look at Sao$_2$

Arterial oxygen saturation (Sao$_2$), expressed as a percentage, represents the actual amount of oxygen bound to Hb divided by the maximum amount of oxygen that could possibly bind to Hb. Because Hb carries most of the blood's oxygen, a normal Sao$_2$ level is 95% to 100%. Pulse oximetry is a noninvasive, real-time estimation of the oxygen saturation of Hb in arterial blood.

How the body responds

The initial response is to increase cardiac output to increase delivery to body tissues as well as to increase the extraction of oxygen from systemic capillaries. In addition, through a slower physiologic process, an increase in hemoglobin levels may also improve oxygen delivery at the cellular level which may have limited benefit to the acutely ill given the speed of the process.

Factors affecting Sao$_2$

Certain conditions impair the body's oxygen supply system, resulting in decreased Sao$_2$, thereby threatening adequate tissue oxygenation. These conditions include those that cause:
• decreased cardiac output, such as heart failure and shock
• inadequate binding of oxygen to Hb, such as carbon monoxide poisoning, nitrate or nitrite therapy, certain anesthetics, and sulfonamide therapy
• severe anemia (inadequate amounts of Hb)
• increased tissue oxygen requirements, such as thyroid storm, malignant hyperthermia, extremely prolonged exercise, delirium tremens, and status epilepticus
• inability of tissue cells to absorb or use the oxygen they receive, such as sepsis, cyanide toxicity, and ethanol toxicity.

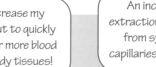

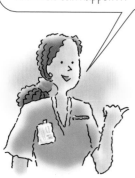

To maintain normal tissue oxygenation and avoid hypoxia, the body needs to compensate for these conditions. Let's see what can happen . . .

I increase my output to quickly deliver more blood to body tissues!

An increased extraction of oxygen from systemic capillaries helps out!

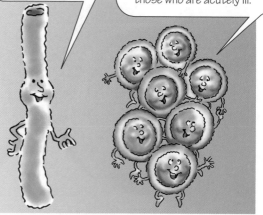

An increased amount of hemoglobin can help, too. However, it might be too slow of a process to benefit those who are acutely ill.

How pulse oximetry works

Performed intermittently or continuously, oximetry is a simple procedure used to monitor arterial oxygen saturation noninvasively. Pulse oximeters usually indicate arterial oxygen saturation values with the symbol *Spo₂*, whereas invasively measured arterial oxygen saturation values are indicated by the symbol *Spo₂*.

In pulse oximetry, two light-emitting diodes (LEDs) send red and infrared light through a pulsating arterial vascular bed such as the one in the fingertip or the earlobe. A photodetector slipped over the finger or earlobe measures the transmitted light as it passes through the vascular bed, detects the relative amount of color absorbed by arterial blood, and provides an estimated arterial oxygen saturation. The accuracy of the reading is dependent on adequate peripheral perfusion to produce an adequate signal.

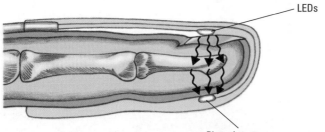

LEDs

Photodetector

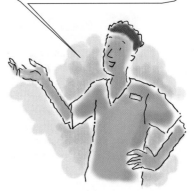

Pulse oximetry can provide an accurate estimate of arterial oxygen saturation without interference from venous blood, skin, tissue—or even bone!

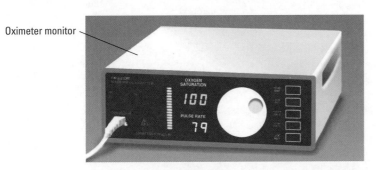

Oximeter monitor

Oximeter cable

Photodetector

Oximeter connector

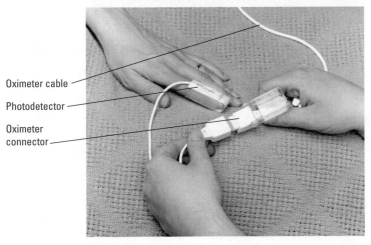

How to use pulse oximetry

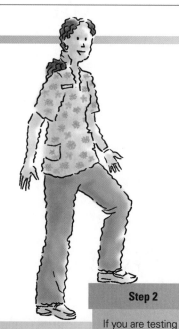

Finger probe

Step 1

Select one finger for the test. Although the index finger is commonly used, a smaller finger may be selected if the patient's fingers are too large for the equipment. Make sure the patient is not wearing false fingernails, and remove nail polish from the test finger. Place the transducer (photodetector) probe over the patient's finger so that light beams and sensors oppose each other. If the patient has long fingernails, position the probe perpendicular to the finger, if possible, or clip the fingernail. Always position the patient's hand at heart level to eliminate venous pulsations and to promote accurate readings.

Step 2

If you are testing a neonate or a small infant, wrap the probe around the foot so that light beams and detectors oppose each other. For a large infant, use a probe that fits on the great toe and secure it to the foot.

Step 3

Turn on the power switch. If the device is working properly, a beep will sound, a display will light momentarily, and the pulse searchlight will flash. The SpO_2 (indicating arterial oxygen saturation by pulse oximetry) and pulse rate displays will show stationary zeros. After four to six heartbeats, the SpO_2 and pulse rate displays will supply information with each beat, and the pulse amplitude indicator will begin tracking the pulse.

Ear probe

Step 1

Following the manufacturer's instructions, attach the ear probe to the patient's earlobe or pinna. Use the ear probe stabilizer for prolonged or exercise testing. Be sure to establish good contact on the ear; an unstable probe may set off the low-perfusion alarm. After the probe has been attached for a few seconds, a saturation reading and pulse waveform will appear on the oximeter's screen.

Step 2

After the procedure, remove the ear probe, turn off and unplug the unit, and clean the probe by gently rubbing it with an alcohol pad.

Step 3

Leave the ear probe in place for 3 or more minutes until readings stabilize at the highest point, or take three separate readings and average them.

Troubleshooting the pulse oximetry system

When using pulse oximetry to measure arterial oxygen saturation, there are several problems that can be avoided or fixed by following good clinical practice. As previously noted, adequate peripheral perfusion is necessary for a reliable reading. Hypothermia and hypotension commonly cause low values as well as elevated bilirubin levels. Falsely high values may result from high carboxyhemoglobin levels or high methemoglobin levels. Intravascular substances, such as lipid emulsions and dyes, acrylic nails, and nail polish may interfere with the sensor as does phototherapy, sunlight, and patient movement.

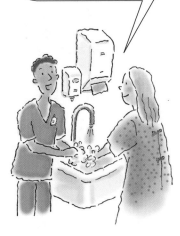

Clean and dry! To maintain a continuous display of arterial oxygen saturation levels, the monitoring site must be clean and dry.

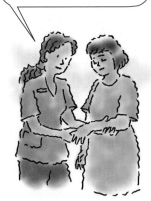

If the skin becomes irritated from adhesives used to keep disposable probes in place, change the oximetry site. You can also replace disposable probes that irritate the skin with nondisposable models.

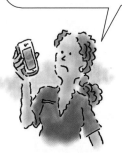

Obtaining a signal can also be a problem with pulse oximeters. If this happens, first check the patient's vital signs. If they are sufficient enough to produce a signal, use the chart below to check for problems and intervene.

Troubleshooting Tips

Problem	Interventions
Poor connection	• Check that the sensors are aligned properly. • Make sure that the wires are intact and fastened securely and that the pulse oximeter is plugged into a power source.
Inadequate or intermittent blood flow to the site	• Check the patient's pulse rate and capillary refill time, and take corrective action if blood flow to the site is decreased. Such action may include loosening restraints, removing tight-fitting clothes, taking off a blood pressure cuff, or checking arterial and IV lines. • If none of these interventions works, find an alternative site. Finding a site with proper circulation may also prove challenging when a patient is receiving vasoconstrictive drugs.
Equipment malfunctions	• Remove the pulse oximeter from the patient, set the alarm limits according to your facility's policies, and try the instrument on yourself or another healthy person. Doing so will tell you whether the equipment is working correctly.

A closer look at $S\bar{v}o_2$

After oxygen is delivered to the tissues, some remains attached to Hb and returns to the heart in venous blood. Mixed venous oxygen saturation ($S\bar{v}o_2$) is the oxygen saturation of Hb in venous blood that returns to the heart from the tissues. Normal $S\bar{v}o_2$ levels are also expressed in percentages, ranging from 60% to 80%. $S\bar{v}o_2$ levels are determined by tissue oxygen consumption and cardiac output (the amount of blood pumped out of the heart per minute).

Arterial blood with oxygen-saturated Hb (normally 96% to 100% saturated) is delivered to body tissues, where cells extract and use about 25% of this oxygen. Then the blood passes into venous circulation, now with Hb only 60% to 80% saturated with oxygen because the cells have taken about 25%. This venous blood is returned to the heart, where $S\bar{v}o_2$ measurements are made in the pulmonary artery.

An alternative to measuring $S\bar{v}o_2$ in the pulmonary artery is central venous monitoring of oxygen saturation ($S\bar{v}o_2$), where a catheter is placed in the superior vena cava or upper right atrium.

In addition, tissue oxygenation saturation (Sto_2), the ratio of oxygenated hemoglobin to total hemoglobin in the microcirculation, can be measured through a noninvasive method. It also assesses the amount of oxygen extraction.

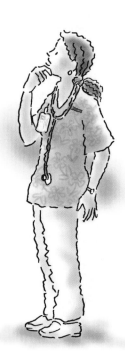

Factors affecting $S\bar{v}o_2$

The patient's $S\bar{v}o_2$ level alone is not useful information. The balance between available oxygen and tissue consumption depends on other factors, such as cardiac output, Sao_2, and Hb levels on the supply side and tissue oxygen needs on the demand side. Any change in the patient's $S\bar{v}o_2$ level typically reflects a change in one or more of these factors.

Abnormal $S\bar{v}o_2$ Levels		
	Conditions that raise $S\bar{v}o_2$ levels and lower the demand for oxygen include: • Anesthesia • chemical paralysis • elevated Sao_2 levels • hypothermiaincreased cardiac output • increased Hb level, and • sedation.	Conditions that lower $S\bar{v}o_2$ levels and raise the demand for oxygen include: • cardiogenic shock • decreased cardiac output • decreased Hb level • hyperthermia/fever • reduced Sao_2 levels • seizures, septic shock, and • shivering.

$S\bar{v}o_2$ monitoring

$S\bar{v}o_2$ monitoring uses a fiberoptic thermodilution pulmonary artery (PA) catheter to continuously monitor oxygen delivery to tissues and oxygen consumption by tissues. Monitoring of $S\bar{v}o_2$ allows rapid detection of impaired oxygen delivery, as from decreased cardiac output, Hb level, or Sao_2. It also helps evaluate a patient's response to drug therapy, endotracheal tube suctioning, ventilator setting changes, positive end-expiratory pressure, and fraction of inspired oxygen.

$Sc\bar{v}o_2$ monitoring

Central venous oxygen saturation ($Sc\bar{v}o_2$) monitoring requires the placement of a central venous catheter with additional fiberoptics and a specialized monitor to continuously monitor venous oxygen saturation.

$Sc\bar{v}o_2$ and $S\bar{v}o_2$ are measurements of the relationship between oxygen consumption and oxygen delivery in the body. $Sc\bar{v}o_2$ values represent regional venous saturations with a normal value of 70%. $Sc\bar{v}o_2$ usually measures slightly higher than $S\bar{v}o_2$ because it has not mixed with the venous blood from the coronary sinus. Although the values may differ, they trend together.

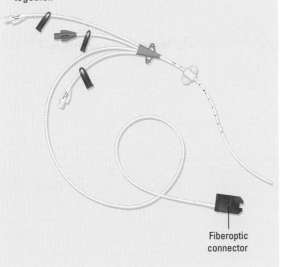

Fiberoptic connector

Sto_2 monitoring

Noninvasive tissue oxygen saturation (Sto_2) monitoring can assist in the early detection of inadequate regional tissue perfusion. It requires a disposable sensor that is placed on the thenar eminence of the hand and a specialized monitor. Near infrared light illuminates the muscle tissue; the returned light produces a measurement of oxygen saturation in the microcirculation.

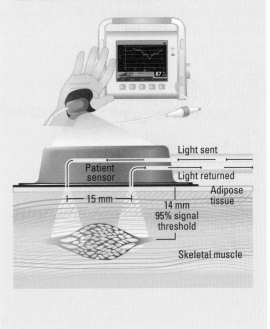

Light sent

Patient sensor

Light returned

15 mm

14 mm 95% signal threshold

Adipose tissue

Skeletal muscle

Troubleshooting the system

If the intensity of the tracing is low:
- ensure that all connections between the catheter and oximeter are secure
- ensure that the catheter is patent and not kinked.
- If the tracing is damped or erratic:
- try to aspirate blood from the catheter to check for patency (if allowed by your facility)
- if you cannot aspirate blood, notify the doctor so that he can replace the catheter
- check the PA waveform to determine whether the catheter has wedged; if the catheter has wedged, turn the patient from side to side and instruct him to cough; if the catheter remains wedged, notify the doctor immediately.

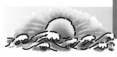

Ride the wave

Normal S$\bar{v}$o$_2$ waveform

This tracing represents a stable, normal S$\bar{v}$o$_2$ level: higher than 60% and lower than 80%. Note the relatively constant line.

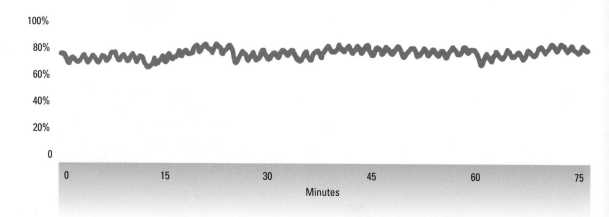

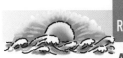

Ride the wave

Abnormal waveforms

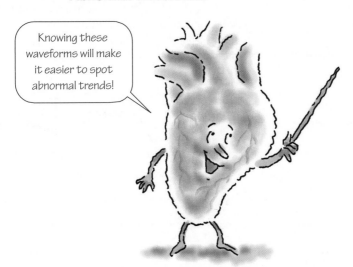

Knowing these waveforms will make it easier to spot abnormal trends!

The first tracing shows a falling venous oxygen saturation Sv̄o₂) level in a patient returning from the operating room after coronary artery bypass surgery. Notice the event marks that indicate atrial pacing and the cardiac index (CI) at about 1 hour, 15 minutes; administration of a vasoactive drug; the patient's plotted response; and his subsequent return to the operating room.

Because a patient's Sv̄o₂ level may change almost immediately after intervention, the subsequent levels can help you determine the intervention's effectiveness. This tracing shows a rise in Sv̄o₂ levels and cardiac output (CO) after the patient has received IV nitroprusside (Nitropress).

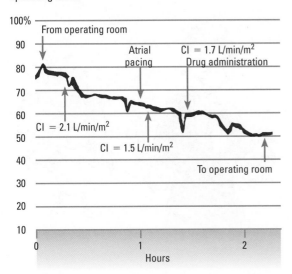

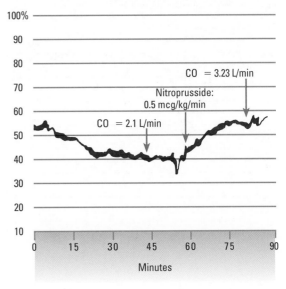

This tracing represents the patient's response to a muscle relaxant.

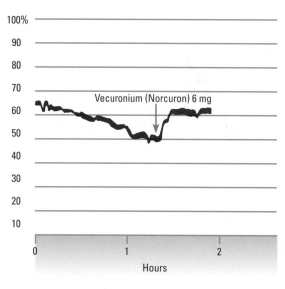

This waveform shows the patient's response to changes in ventilator settings. Note that increasing the positive end-expiratory pressure (PEEP) causes an increase in $S\bar{v}o_2$; therefore, the fraction of inspired oxygen (Fio_2) can be decreased.

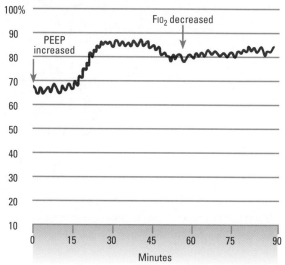

This waveform shows typical changes in the $S\bar{v}o_2$ level as a result of various activities.

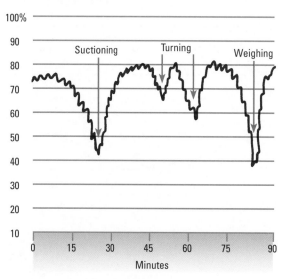

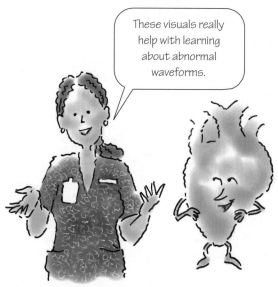

These visuals really help with learning about abnormal waveforms.

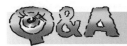

Show and tell

Identify the names of the S$\bar{v}o_2$ waveforms shown in these illustrations.

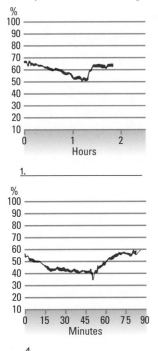

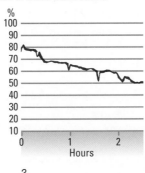

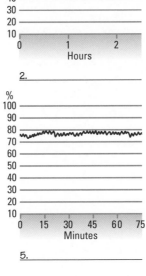

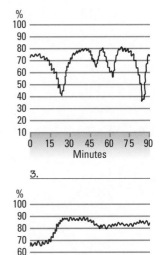

1. _____

2. _____

3. _____

4. _____

5. _____

6. _____

Matchmaker

Match the abbreviations with the correct spelled-out version for each.

1. Dao_2 _____   **A.** partial pressure of arterial oxygen

2. Sao_2 _____   **B.** arterial oxygen delivery

3. $S\bar{v}o_2$ _____   **C.** venous oxygen reserve

4. Pao_2 _____   **D.** arterial oxygen saturation

5. Rvo_2 _____   **E.** mixed venous oxygen saturation

Answers: Show and tell: 1. Patient response to a muscle relaxant, 2. Falling S$\bar{v}o_2$ level, 3. Typical changes in the S$\bar{v}o_2$ level as a result of various activities, 4. Rise in S$\bar{v}o_2$ levels and cardiac output, 5. Normal S$\bar{v}o_2$ waveform, 6. Patient response to change in ventilator settings. *Matchmaker:* 1. B, 2. D, 3. E, 4. A, 5. C.

Suggested References

Alspach, J.G. (Ed.). *Core Curriculum for Critical Care Nursing*, 6th ed. Philadelphia: W.B. Saunders Co., 2006.

American Thoracic Society. *Measuring Oxygenation*. Retrieved January 18, 2015, from http://www.thoracic.org/clinical/copd-guidelines/for-health-professionals/management-of-stable-copd/long-term/oxygen-therapy/measuring-oxygenation.php.

Carlson, K.K. (Ed.). *AACN Advanced Critical Care Nursing*. Philadelphia: Elsevier, 2009.

Foster, C., et al. (Eds.). *Washington Manual of Medical Therapeutics*, 33rd ed. Philadelphia: Lippincott Williams & Wilkins, 2010, 268–271.

Lippincott's Nursing Procedures & Skills. Philadelphia: Lippincott Williams & Wilkins, 2009. Accessed via the online program on September 1, 2009.

McLauglin, M.A. (Ed.). *Cardiovascular Care Made Incredibly Easy*, 3rd ed. Philadelphia: Lippincott Williams & Wilkins, 2014.

Morton, P.G., and Fontaine, D.K. *Critical Care Nursing: A Holistic Approach*, 9th ed. Philadelphia: Lippincott Williams & Wilkins, 2009.

Weigand, D.L., and Carlson, K.K. *AACN Procedure Manual for Critical Care*, 6th ed. St. Louis: Elsevier Saunders, 2010.

Woods, S., et al. *Cardiac Nursing*, 6th ed. Philadelphia: Lippincott Williams & Wilkins, 2010.

Chapter 9

Minimally invasive hemodynamic monitoring

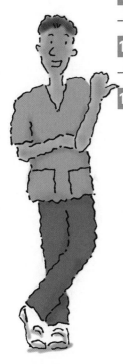

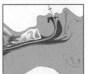
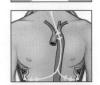

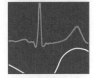
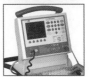

Understanding minimally invasive hemodynamic monitoring

Although invasive hemodynamic monitoring using a pulmonary artery (PA) catheter remains the gold standard for clinical practice, minimally invasive monitoring techniques are proving to be reliable, safe options that yield results that relate with PA catheter readings.

Minimally invasive hemodynamic monitoring techniques are easier to use, can be applied in many clinical settings, and provide reproducible results.

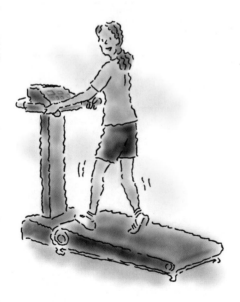

Esophageal Doppler hemodynamic monitoring

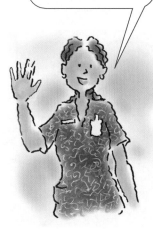

Esophageal Doppler hemodynamic monitoring can keep track of five hemodynamic values—not bad for a minimally invasive monitoring system!

Esophageal Doppler hemodynamic monitoring is a minimally invasive method of using ultrasound to measure heart function. It involves placement of a probe into the esophagus. By measuring blood flow through the heart valves or ventricular outflow tracts, this monitoring system can monitor:

- cardiac output (CO)
- stroke volume (SV)
- cardiac index (CI)
- systemic vascular resistance
- systemic vascular resistance index.

Indications and contraindications

This type of monitoring is appropriate for:

☑ sedated, critically ill patients with difficult fluid management

☑ use during and after cardiac surgery

☑ patients undergoing major or high-risk surgery or high-risk patients undergoing any surgery excluding head, neck, and esophageal surgery

☑ patients treated in critical care requiring cardiac output monitoring for any reason

It is not recommended for patients:

☒ undergoing intra-aortic balloon pump (IABP) counterpulsation

☒ with severe coarctation of the aorta

☒ with a disorder of the pharynx, esophagus, or stomach

☒ with carcinoma of the esophagus or pharynx or previous esophageal surgery, esophageal stricture, varices, or pharyngeal pouch

☒ with a bleeding disorder

☒ with severe coagulopathies

Pros and cons of esophageal Doppler hemodynamic monitoring

Pros	Cons
• It is minimally invasive. • Easier to insert with rare complications.	• It is difficult to align the ultrasound beam with the flow of blood. (If the beam is not properly angled, the results are not reliable.) • It carries the risk of esophageal damage or perforation. • The patient may require sedation because of the stiffness of the probe.

Transducer probe placement

Transducer probe placement for esophageal Doppler hemodynamic monitoring is similar to inserting a nasogastric or orogastric tube, and typically can be performed by a nurse at the bedside. However, the patient usually requires sedation for this procedure because the probe is rigid.

The stiff probe is lubricated and then inserted nasally or orally to a depth of 14" to 16" (35.5 to 40.5 cm). Each probe has depth markers to demonstrate appropriate depth placement. The probe can be taped in place or left unsecured to allow for adjustments (if the patient is sedated). When the probe is positioned properly, it is ready to measure blood flow in the descending thoracic aorta.

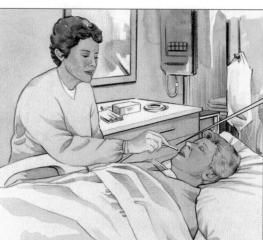

First, the transducer probe is lubricated. It can then be inserted nasally or orally. Oral placement is shown here.

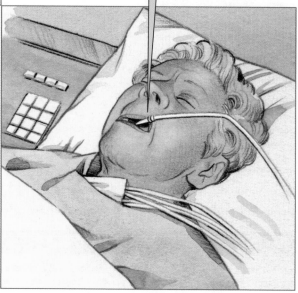

Depth markers on the probe enable easy insertion to a depth of 35.5 to 40.5 cm.

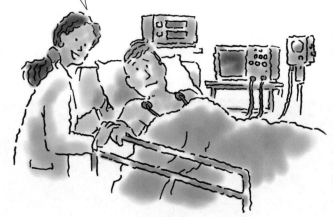

The nurse can typically perform the insertion of a transducer probe. However, the patient usually requires sedation.

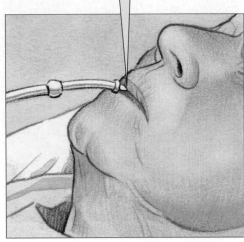

The probe can then be secured with tape or left unsecured (if the patient is sedated).

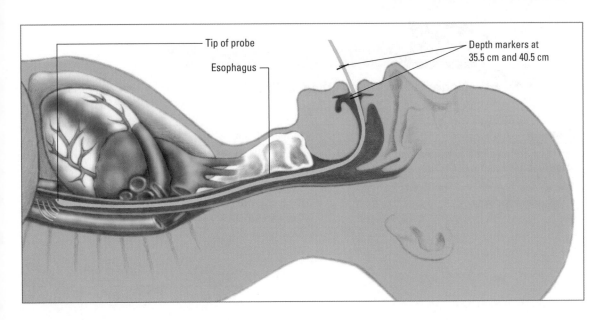

Tip of probe

Esophagus

Depth markers at 35.5 cm and 40.5 cm

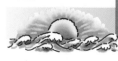

Ride the wave

Esophageal Doppler hemodynamic monitoring waveform

This normal waveform shows good capture of blood flow. Key aspects of the waveform include peak velocity and systolic blood flow in seconds corrected for heart rate (HR).

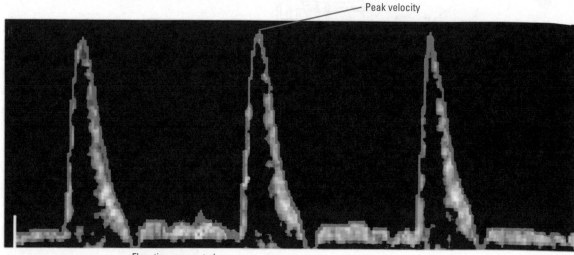

Peak velocity

Flow time, corrected ⟶

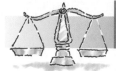

On the level

Normal values in esophageal Doppler hemodynamic monitoring

Parameter	Normal values
Flow time, corrected (the time in seconds of systolic blood flow, corrected to heart rate)	330 to 360 milliseconds
Peak velocity (the velocity of the blood measured at the peak of systole)	20 years: 90 to 120 cm/sec 50 years: 60 to 90 cm/sec 70 years: 50 to 80 cm/sec

A closer look at the monitoring system

This monitor automatically measures such values as heart rate, peak velocity (PV), flow time corrected (FTc), and more. Other hemodynamic monitoring parameters are then derived from these direct measurements, including CO, CI, SV, stroke volume index, and systemic vascular resistance.

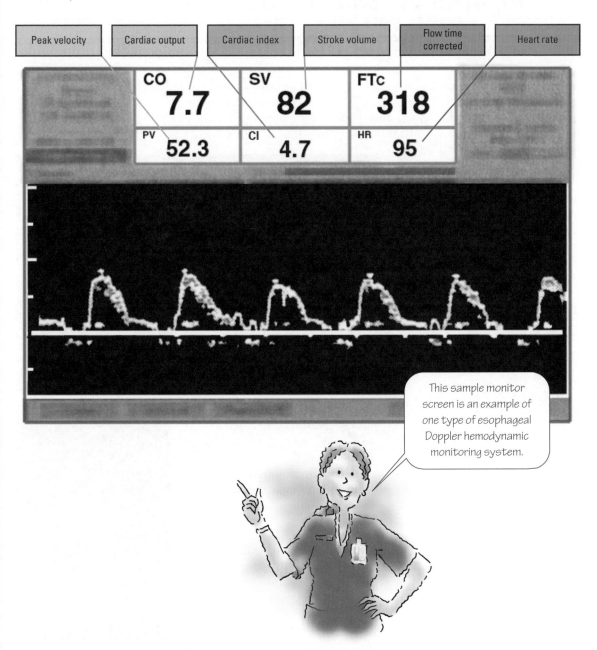

| Peak velocity | Cardiac output | Cardiac index | Stroke volume | Flow time corrected | Heart rate |

CO 7.7   SV 82   FTc 318

PV 52.3   CI 4.7   HR 95

This sample monitor screen is an example of one type of esophageal Doppler hemodynamic monitoring system.

Arterial pressure-based cardiac output monitoring

Arterial pressure-based cardiac output (APCO) monitoring provides a minimally invasive method to measure CO, which is SV multiplied by the patient's HR. In APCO monitoring, pulse pressure (systolic blood pressure [SBP] minus diastolic blood pressure [DBP]) is proportional to SV with variability in the arterial pressure identified as a standard deviation (SD).

APCO uses a patient's existing arterial catheter to continuously calculate and display CO. The arterial waveform is analyzed by one of three methods to track changes in stroke volume and CO. All methods use a different clinically validated algorithm to determine the patient's CO.

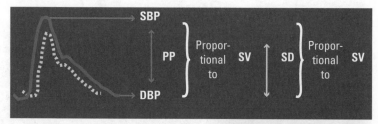

1 **Pulse flow and pressure analysis:** uses pulse contour and pulse power analysis; incorporates an SD of the full waveform to measure SV.

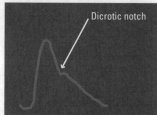

2 **Pulse contour analysis:** measures and monitors SV on a beat-to-beat basis looking at the morphology of the arterial waveform from the beginning of systole to the dicrotic notch.

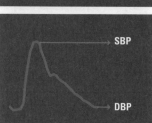

3 **Pulse power analysis:** looks at the power of the whole pulse—systolic and diastolic; does not look at beat morphology.

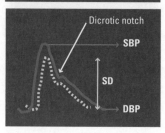

A closer look at APCO

The arterial catheter and line are connected to a sensor, transducer, and specialized monitor preprogrammed with the clinically validated algorithm for determining CO.

Three devices are currently available. One system requires that the patient's age, gender, height, and weight be entered into the computer but no external calibration. Two others require an external calibration method. APCO is very useful in helping to determine a patient's fluid status and his potential response to a fluid challenge before he has significant changes in blood pressure.

Radial artery catheter

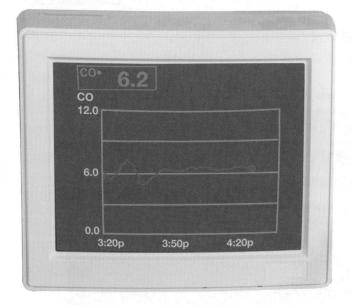

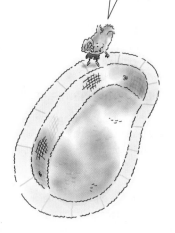

I don't like the looks of this fluid status!

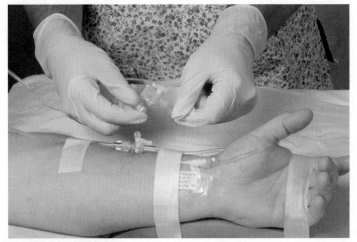

Interfering factors for APCO

- incorrect leveling of transducer and sensor
- incorrect zeroing
- IABP
- arrhythmias
- artificial heart or ventricular assist device
- dampened pressure waveforms
- air bubbles in the fluid line
- limitations of APCO monitoring: less accurate with changes in vascular tone and reactivity

Impedance cardiography

Impedance cardiography provides a noninvasive alternative for tracking hemodynamic status. This technique provides information about a patient's cardiac index, preload, afterload, contractility, cardiac output, and blood flow by measuring low-level electricity that flows harmlessly through the body from electrodes placed on the patient's thorax. These electrodes detect signals elicited from the changing volume and velocity of blood flow through the aorta. The signals are interpreted by the impedance monitor as a waveform. Cardiac output is computed from this waveform and the electrocardiogram.

Benefits of impedance cardiography

Impedance cardiography monitoring eliminates the risk of infection, bleeding, pneumothorax, emboli, and arrhythmias associated with traditional invasive hemodynamic monitoring. The accuracy of results obtained by this method is comparable to that obtained by thermodilution. In addition, the impedance cardiography monitor automatically updates information every second to tenth heartbeat, providing real-time data.

Monitoring equipment for impedance cardiography

To begin impedance cardiography, assemble the impedance cardiography monitor, printer, and disposable sensors.

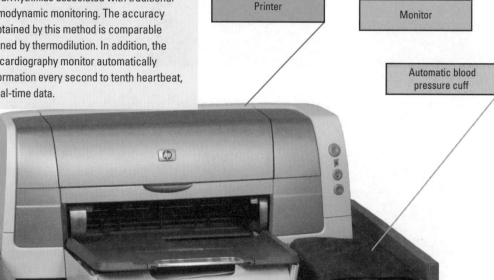

Printer

Monitor

Automatic blood pressure cuff

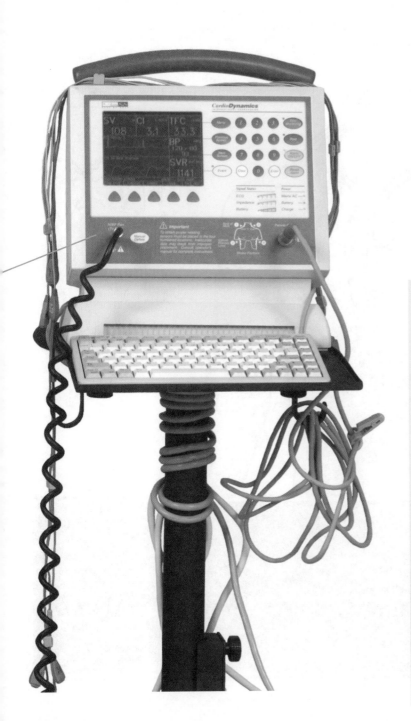

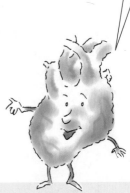

Impedance cardiography is harmless and noninvasive. So there's nothing to *impede* you from using it.

Indications for impedance cardiography

Impedance cardiography helps monitor patients who would have a high risk of complications from thermodilution methods. Because of its portability, the impedance cardiography unit may be used in the operating room, postanesthesia care unit, and intensive care unit.

However, baseline impedance cardiography values may be reduced in patients who have conditions characterized by increased fluid in the chest, such as pulmonary edema and pulmonary effusion. Also, impedance cardiography values may be lower than thermodilution values in patients with tachycardia and other arrhythmias.

Impedance cardiography electrode placement

This illustration shows proper placement of the four pairs of electrodes needed for impedance cardiography. This system uses a low-voltage current to detect resistance (impedance) to the current between electrodes.

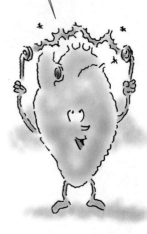

Impedance cardiography uses a low-voltage electric current to detect resistance, or impedance, to the current between the electrodes.

Outer electrodes transmit current

Inner electrodes detect impedance

Memory board

Currents and resistance

Picture a stream when you think about impedance cardiography electrode placement.

Preparing the patient for impedance cardiography

To prepare a patient for impedance cardiography, first help him into the proper position. He should be supine, with the head of the bed elevated at or below 20 degrees. Clean the skin on each side of his neck and on both sides of his chest at the midaxillary line directly across from the xiphoid process with some gauze and warm water. Shaving may be necessary to promote adhesion of the electrodes.

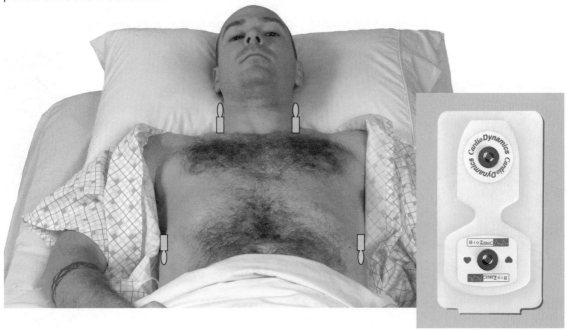

Next, hold the patient cable so that the torso diagram is upright and facing you.

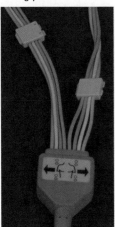

Connect the leads from top to bottom, following the "BPGO" order:

- blue
- purple
- green
- orange

Then attach the blood pressure cuff to the patient's arm.

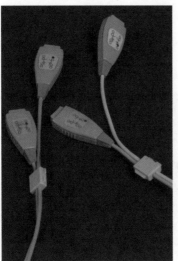

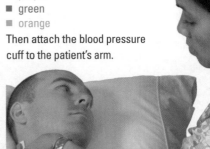

Using the impedance cardiography monitor

To use the impedance cardiography monitor, plug it in and turn on the power. The welcome display screen should appear. If necessary, enter the basic patient data as prompted by the monitor. The START MONITORING screen should appear.

Before initiating monitoring, advise your patient to remain still. Then press the START MONITOR key. Evaluate the signal strength on the screen to make sure that at least three green lights appear on the impedance cardiography and electrocardiogram (ECG) signal bars. A beep should also be audible as each R wave appears on the ECG screen.

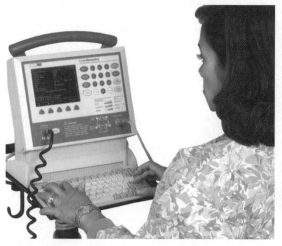

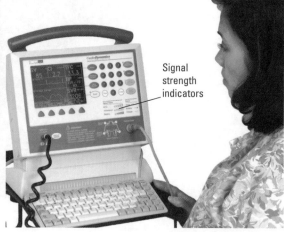

Signal strength indicators

Lastly, note the waveforms and values on the monitor and document the values by printing a report.

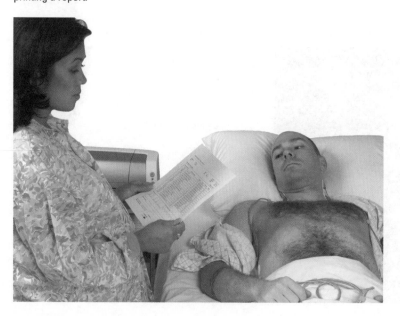

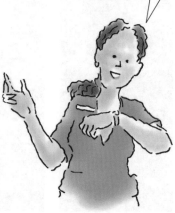

Electrodes should be replaced every 24 hours during continuous impedance cardiography monitoring.

Understanding hemodynamic indices

After you connect your patient to an impedance cardiography monitor, you can easily obtain the hemodynamic data needed to determine his stability and plan treatment and care. With an impedance cardiography monitoring unit, you can measure these values:

cardiac index (CI): cardiac output (CO) divided by body surface area, which puts CO in perspective for the patient's size

cardiac output (CO): the volume of blood pumped through the heart (measured in L/min)

dZ/dt: indicator of peak flow

ejection fraction (EF): volume of blood ejected from the left ventricle in a single myocardial contraction (expressed as a percentage)

end-diastolic volume (EDV): volume of blood in the left ventricle at the end of diastole; also known as the *preload volume* (measured in milliliters)

heart rate (HR): number of heartbeats in 1 minute

left cardiac work index (LCWI): reflection of myocardial oxygen consumption

preejection period (PEP): time between the onset of ventricular activity and the opening of the aortic valve (measured in seconds)

stroke volume (SV): amount of blood pumped from the ventricle with each myocardial contraction (measured in milliliters)

systemic vascular resistance (SVR): resistance against which the left ventricle pumps

ventricular ejection time (VET): amount of time that blood is flowing out of the ventricles

Zo: base impedance, or the amount of resistance met by the electric current passing through the thorax.

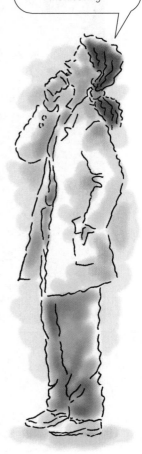

Look at all these indices! Just shows how valuable a tool impedance cardiography is for hemodynamic monitoring!

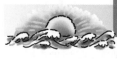

Understanding the impedance cardiography waveform

A waveform produced by an arterial pressure monitoring system is based on pressure. Although a waveform produced by impedance cardiography is similar, it is based on the volume and velocity of aortic blood flow. It captures the electrical impedance of pulsatile flow that is generated by every heartbeat. The components of an impedance cardiography waveform are shown below.

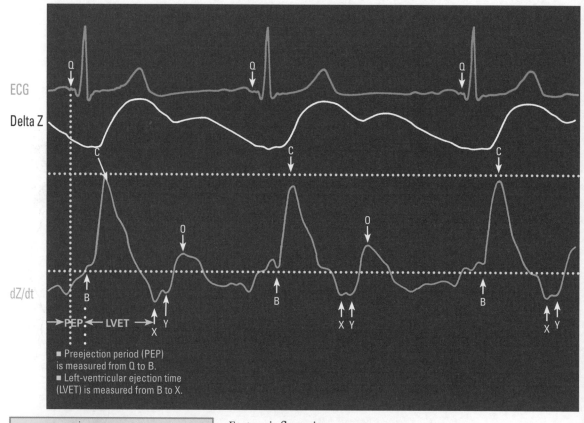

- Preejection period (PEP) is measured from Q to B.
- Left-ventricular ejection time (LVET) is measured from B to X.

Key

Q = Start of ventricular depolarization
B = Opening of pulmonic and aortic valve
C = Maximal deflection
X = Closure of aortic valve
Y = Closure of pulmonic valve
O = Mitral opening snap/rapid filling of ventricles

Factors influencing correct measurements
1. Incorrect lead placement
2. Incorrect patient positioning
3. Arrhythmias such as atrial fibrillation
4. Weight >351lb
5. Acute aortic insufficiency
6. Advanced sepsis
7. IABP
8. Extreme tachycardia

Ultrasound cardiac output measurement

Ultrasound cardiac output measurement (USCOM), a new technology developed by USCOM Limited, uses continuous wave Doppler ultrasound to evaluate heart function. This entirely noninvasive system directs the Doppler ultrasound at two anatomic areas:

1. the suprasternal notch to evaluate the left side of the heart by looking at aortic valve blood flow

2. the left sternal edge to evaluate the right side of the heart by looking at pulmonic valve blood flow.
Parameters measured by USCOM include CO, CI, SV, HR, velocity time integral, minute distance, ejection time percent, peak flow velocity, and mean pressure gradient.

USCOM monitor

This illustration displays the work screen of an ultrasound cardiac output measurement (USCOM) monitor. This monitoring system is produced by USCOM Limited.

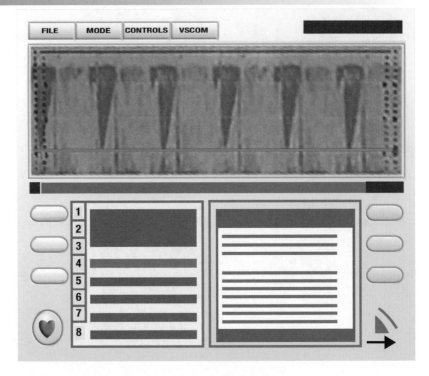

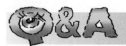

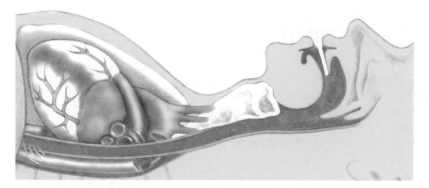

Color my world

Use a green pen or pencil to trace the proper placement of an esophageal Doppler probe in the illustration.

Picture imperfect

Identify the picture that shows correct electrode placement for impedance cardiography.

1.

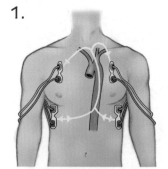

2.

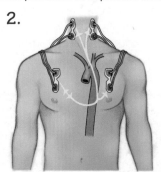

3.

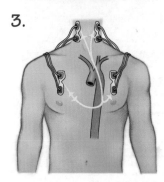

4.

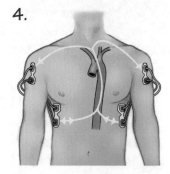

Answers: Color my world: After lubricating the tube, insert it either nasally or orally to the appropriate depth marker. The tip of the probe should lie in the esophagus, posterior to the heart. Picture imperfect: Correct electrode placement is shown in #3.

Suggested References

Foster, C., et al. (Eds.). *Washington Manual of Medical Therapeutics*, 33rd ed. Philadelphia: Lippincott, Williams, & Wilkins, 2010, 268–271.

Marik PE. "Noninvasive Cardiac Output Monitors: A State of Art Review," *Journal of Cardiothoracic and Vascular Anesthesia* 27(1):121–134, Feb 2013.

Program, A.T. *Esophageal Doppler Ultrasound-Based Cardiac Output Monitoring For Real-time Therapeutic Management of Hospitalized Patients: A Review*. Rockville: Agency for Healthcare Research and Quality, 2007.

Schober, P. "Transesophageal Doppler Devices: A Technical Review," *Journal of Clinical Monitoring and Computing* 391–401, 2009.

Chapter 10

Circulatory assist devices

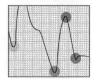

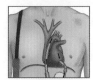

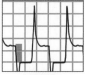

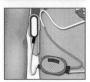

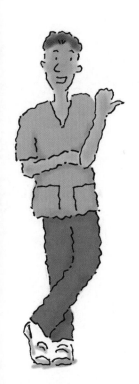

Understanding circulatory assist devices

Circulatory assist devices support or aid the heart's pumping ability in patients with heart failure. These devices improve blood flow to the myocardium and the rest of the body while reducing myocardial workload.

Such devices include intra-aortic balloon pump (IABP) counterpulsation, ventricular assist devices (VADs), and extracorporeal membrane oxygenation (ECMO).

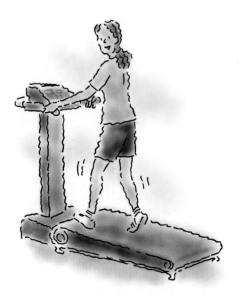

IABP counterpulsation

Providing temporary support for the heart's left ventricle, IABP counterpulsation mechanically displaces blood within the aorta by means of an intra-aortic balloon attached to an external pump console. The balloon is usually inserted through the common femoral artery and positioned with its tip just distal to the left subclavian artery. When used correctly, IABP improves two key aspects of myocardial physiology: it increases the supply of oxygen-rich blood to the myocardium and decreases myocardial oxygen demand.

Insertion of the intra-aortic balloon

The provider may insert the balloon percutaneously through the femoral or subclavian artery into the descending thoracic aorta, using a modified Seldinger technique.

Indications for IABP counterpulsation

Intra-aortic balloon pump (IABP) counterpulsation is recommended for patients with:
- refractory anginas
- ventricular arrhythmias associated with ischemia
- pump failure caused by cardiogenic shock, intraoperative myocardial infarction (MI), or low cardiac output after bypass surgery
- low cardiac output secondary to acute mechanical defects after MI (such as ventricular septal defect, papillary muscle rupture, or left ventricular aneurysm)
- a suspected high-grade lesion (used perioperatively for those who are undergoing such procedures as angioplasty, thrombolytic therapy, cardiac surgery, and cardiac catheterization).

IABP counterpulsation is contraindicated in patients with:
- severe aortic insufficiency
- aortic aneurysm
- severe peripheral vascular disease.

Step 1
First, the provider accesses the vessel with an 18G angiography needle and removes the inner stylet.

Step 2
Then, he passes the guide wire through the needle and removes the needle.

Step 3
After passing a #8 to #10.5 French vessel dilator over the guide wire into the vessel, he removes the vessel dilator, leaving the guide wire in place.

Step 4
The doctor then passes an introducer (dilator and sheath assembly) over the guide wire into the vessel until about 1″ (2.5 cm) remains above the insertion site. He then removes the inner dilator, leaving the introducer sheath and guide wire in place.

Step 5
After passing the balloon over the guide wire into the introducer sheath, the doctor advances the catheter into position, ⅜″ to ¾″ (1 to 2 cm) distal to the left subclavian artery under fluoroscopic guidance.

Step 6
He attaches the balloon to the control system to initiate counterpulsation. The balloon catheter then unfurls.

Surgical insertion sites for the intra-aortic balloon

If an intra-aortic balloon cannot be inserted percutaneously, the provider will insert it surgically, using a femoral or transthoracic approach.

Femoral approach	Subclavian approach	Transthoracic approach
Insertion through the femoral artery requires a cutdown and an arteriotomy. The doctor passes the balloon through a Dacron graft that has been sewn to the artery.	Insertion through the subclavian artery is done under fluoroscopic guidance; the balloon wire is positioned in the descending thoracic aorta and the balloon is inserted and placed into an appropriate position.	If femoral insertion is unsuccessful, the doctor may use a transthoracic approach. He inserts the balloon in an antegrade direction through the subclavian artery and then positions it in the descending thoracic aorta.

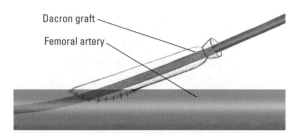

Dacron graft

Femoral artery

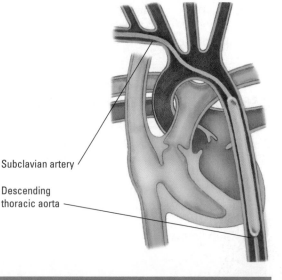

Subclavian artery

Descending thoracic aorta

How the intra-aortic balloon pump works

Made of polyurethane, the intra-aortic balloon is attached to an external pump console by means of a large-lumen catheter. The illustrations here show the direction of blood flow when the pump inflates and deflates the balloon.

Balloon inflation	Balloon deflation
The balloon inflates as the aortic valve closes and diastole begins. During diastole, the balloon inflates sending blood back to the heart which then increases perfusion to the coronary arteries.	The balloon deflates before ventricular ejection, when the aortic valve opens. This deflation permits ejection of blood from the left ventricle against a lowered resistance. As a result, aortic end-diastolic pressure and afterload decrease and cardiac output rises.

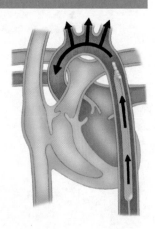

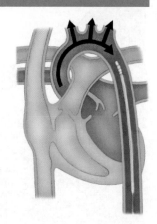

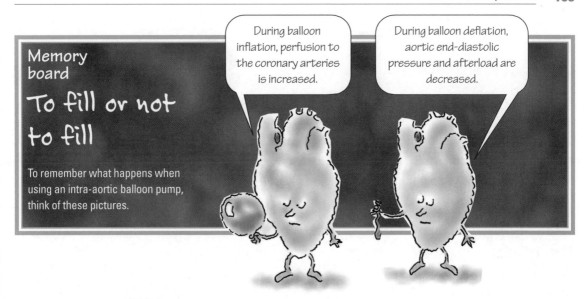

During balloon inflation, perfusion to the coronary arteries is increased.

During balloon deflation, aortic end-diastolic pressure and afterload are decreased.

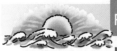

Ride the wave

Interpreting IABP waveforms

During IABP counterpulsation, you can use electrocardiogram (ECG) and arterial pressure waveforms to determine whether the balloon pump is functioning properly.

Normal inflation–deflation timing

Balloon inflation occurs after aortic valve closure; deflation occurs during isovolumetric contraction, just before the aortic valve opens. In a properly timed waveform such as this one, the inflation point lies at or slightly above the dicrotic notch. Both inflation and deflation cause a sharp V. Peak diastolic pressure exceeds peak systolic pressure; peak systolic pressure exceeds assisted peak systolic pressure.

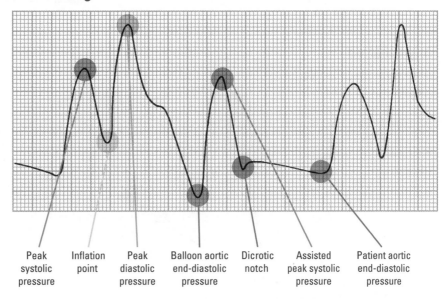

Peak systolic pressure

Inflation point

Peak diastolic pressure

Balloon aortic end-diastolic pressure

Dicrotic notch

Assisted peak systolic pressure

Patient aortic end-diastolic pressure

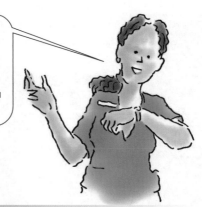

With IABP, timing is everything. Early or late inflation or deflation can endanger the patient. Check out these waveforms to learn how to spot IABP problems!

Early inflation

With early inflation, the inflation point lies before the dicrotic notch. Early inflation dangerously increases myocardial stress and decreases cardiac output.

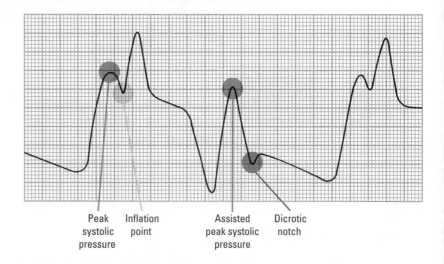

Peak systolic pressure   Inflation point   Assisted peak systolic pressure   Dicrotic notch

Early deflation

With early deflation, a U shape appears and peak systolic pressure is less than or equal to assisted peak systolic pressure. Early deflation won't decrease afterload or myocardial oxygen consumption.

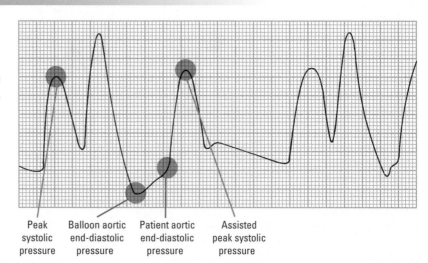

Peak systolic pressure   Balloon aortic end-diastolic pressure   Patient aortic end-diastolic pressure   Assisted peak systolic pressure

Late inflation

With late inflation, the dicrotic notch precedes the inflation point, and the notch and the inflation point create a W shape. Late inflation can lead to a reduction in peak diastolic pressure, coronary and systemic perfusion augmentation time, and augmented coronary perfusion pressure.

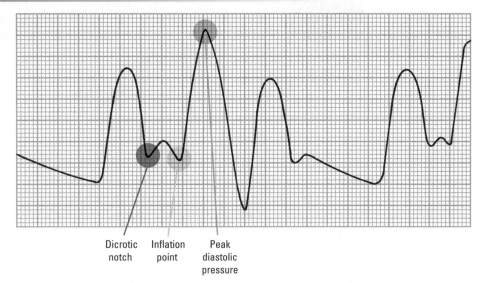

Dicrotic notch Inflation point Peak diastolic pressure

Late deflation

With late deflation, peak systolic pressure exceeds assisted peak systolic pressure. Late deflation puts the patient at risk by increasing afterload, myocardial oxygen consumption, cardiac workload, and preload.

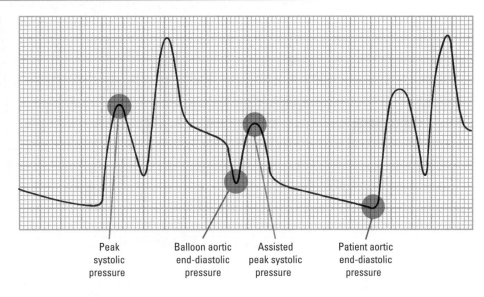

Peak systolic pressure Balloon aortic end-diastolic pressure Assisted peak systolic pressure Patient aortic end-diastolic pressure

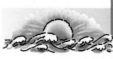

Heart rate and blood pressure effects on IABP waveforms

Changes in heart rate and blood pressure cause changes in the width and height of the balloon pressure plateau of the IABP waveform, as shown in these illustrations.

Changes in heart rate

Variations in heart rate affect the width of the balloon pressure plateau. *Note:* If the width of the balloon pressure plateau is not consistent with the patient's heart rate, there may be a significant error in timing.

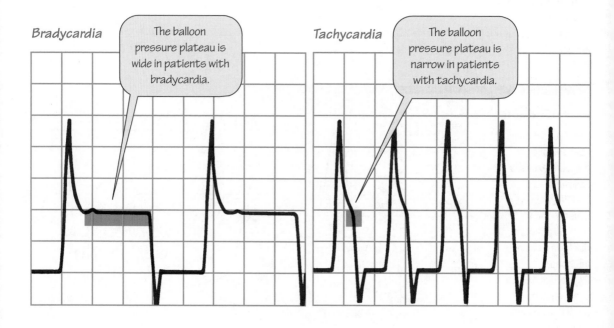

Bradycardia

The balloon pressure plateau is wide in patients with bradycardia.

Tachycardia

The balloon pressure plateau is narrow in patients with tachycardia.

Changes in blood pressure

Variations in blood pressure affect the height of the balloon pressure plateau.

Hypotension

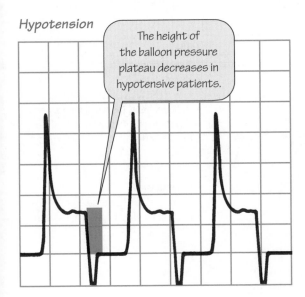

The height of the balloon pressure plateau decreases in hypotensive patients.

Hypertension

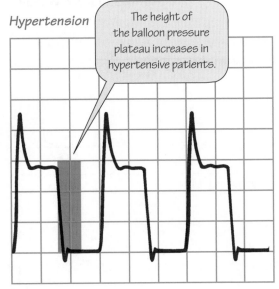

The height of the balloon pressure plateau increases in hypertensive patients.

Complications of IABP counterpulsation

IABP counterpulsation may cause numerous complications. The most common—arterial embolism—stems from clot formation on the balloon surface. Other potential complications include extension or rupture of an aortic aneurysm, visceral and limb ischemia, femoral or iliac artery perforation, femoral artery occlusion, and sepsis. Bleeding at the insertion site may result from pump-induced thrombocytopenia.

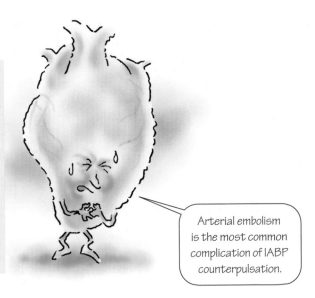

Arterial embolism is the most common complication of IABP counterpulsation.

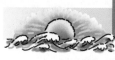

Abnormal IABP waveforms

Abnormality	Waveform	Causes
Low balloon pressure plateau		• Hypotension • Hypovolemia • Low systemic vascular resistance • Balloon that is too small for the aorta or low balloon inflation volume • Positioning of balloon too low in aorta
High balloon pressure plateau		• Hypertension • Balloon that is too large for the aorta • Restriction of gas flow in the system
Balloon pressure baseline elevation		• Restriction of gas flow • Overpressurized gas in system
Balloon pressure baseline depression		• Helium leak • Inappropriate timing settings • Mechanical defect

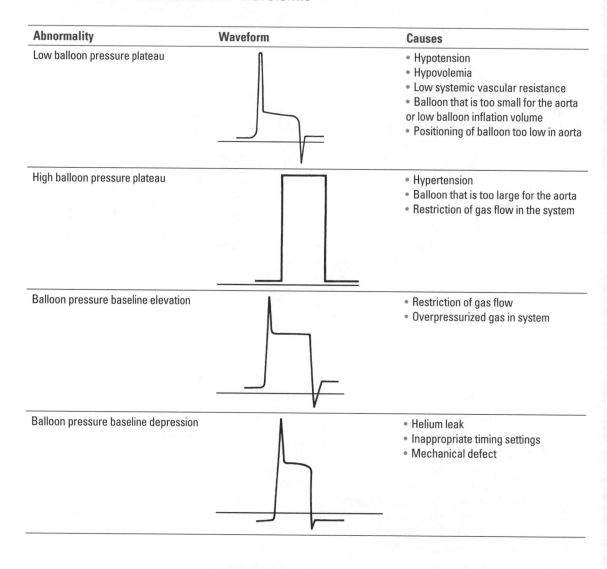

Troubleshooting an IABP

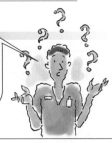

Wondering what to do if there's a problem with an IABP? Well, we've got the answers for you!

Problem	Possible causes	Interventions
High gas leak (automatic mode only)	Balloon leakage or abrasion	• Check for blood in the tubing. • Stop pumping. • Notify the doctor to remove the balloon.
	Condensation in extension tubing, volume limiter disk, or both	• Remove condensate from the tubing and volume limiter disk. • Refill, autopurge, and resume pumping.
	Kink in balloon catheter or tubing	• Check the catheter and tubing for kinks and loose connections; straighten and tighten any found. • Refill and resume pumping.
	Tachycardia	• Change wean control to 1:2 or operate on "manual" mode. • Autopurge the balloon every 1 to 2 hours, and monitor the balloon pressure waveform closely.
	Malfunctioning or loose volume limiter disk	• Replace or tighten the disk. • Refill, autopurge, and resume pumping.
	System leak	• Perform a leak test.
Balloon line block (in automatic mode only)	Kink in balloon or catheter	• Check the catheter and tubing for kinks and loose connections; straighten and tighten any found. • Refill and resume pumping.
	Balloon catheter not unfurled; sheath or balloon positioned too high	• Notify the doctor immediately to verify placement. • Anticipate the need for repositioning or manual inflation of the balloon.
	Condensation in tubing, volume limiter disk, or both	• Remove condensate from the tubing and volume limiter disk. • Refill, autopurge, and resume pumping.
	Balloon too large for aorta	• Decrease volume control percentage by one notch.
	Malfunctioning volume limiter disk or incorrect volume limiter disk size	• Replace the volume limiter disk. • Refill, autopurge, and resume pumping.
No electrocardiogram (ECG) trigger	Inadequate signal	• Adjust ECG gain, and change the lead or trigger mode.
	Lead disconnected	• Replace the lead.
	Improper ECG input mode (skin or monitor) selected	• Adjust ECG input to appropriate mode (skin or monitor).

Continued...

Problem	Possible causes	Interventions
No atrial pressure trigger	Arterial line damped	• Flush the line.
	Arterial line open to atmosphere	• Check connections on the arterial pressure line.
Trigger mode change	Trigger mode changed while pumping	• Resume pumping.
Irregular heart rhythm	Patient experiencing arrhythmia, such as atrial fibrillation or ectopic beats	• Change to R or QRS sense (if necessary to accommodate irregular rhythm). • Notify the doctor of arrhythmia.
Erratic atrioventricular (AV) pacing	Demand for paced rhythm occurring when in AV sequential trigger mode	• Change to pacer reject trigger or QRS sense.
Noisy ECG signal	Malfunctioning leads	• Replace the leads. • Check the ECG cable.
	Electrocautery in use	• Switch to atrial pressure trigger.
Internal trigger	Trigger mode set on internal 80 beats/min	• Select an alternative trigger if the patient has a heartbeat or rhythm. • Keep in mind that the internal trigger is used only during cardiopulmonary bypass or cardiac arrest.
Purge incomplete	OFF button pressed during autopurge; interrupted purge cycle	• Initiate autopurging again, or initiate pumping.
High fill pressure	Malfunctioning volume limiter disk	• Replace the volume limiter disk. • Refill, autopurge, and resume pumping.
	Occluded vent line or valve	• Attempt to resume pumping. • If unsuccessful, notify the doctor and contact the manufacturer.
No balloon drive	No volume limiter disk	• Insert the volume limiter disk, and lock it securely in place.
	Tubing disconnected	• Reconnect the tubing. • Refill, autopurge, and pump.
Incorrect timing	INFLATE and DEFLATE controls set incorrectly	• Place the INFLATE and DEFLATE controls at set midpoints. • Reassess timing and readjust.
Low volume percentage	Volume control percentage not 100%	• Assess the cause of decreased volume, and reset (if necessary).

Ventricular assist devices

A VAD is implanted to provide support to a failing heart. The device consists of a blood pump, cannulas, and a pneumatic or electrical drive console (or controller). A VAD can provide systemic and pulmonary support.

VADs are designed to decrease the heart's workload and increase cardiac output in patients with ventricular failure. They are commonly used as a bridge to cardiac transplantation. VADs are also indicated for use in patients with:

- end-stage heart failure, but who are ineligible for a transplant (Destination Therapy)
- cardiogenic shock that does not respond to maximal pharmacologic therapy
- inability to be weaned from cardiopulmonary bypass.

Left VAD

Pulsatile pump

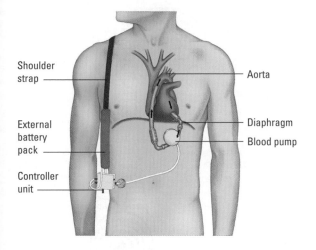

Shoulder strap

Aorta

External battery pack

Diaphragm

Blood pump

Controller unit

Continous flow pump

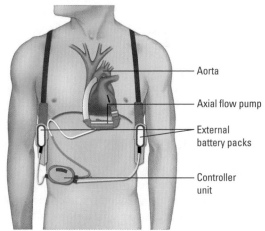

Aorta

Axial flow pump

External battery packs

Controller unit

Procedure

Insertion of a VAD involves a specific surgical procedure, in which blood is diverted from a ventricle to an artificial pump. The diversion is created by inserting a cannula into either the atria or ventricles that directs blood to the pump. This pump then functions as the ventricle.

Implantable VADs

The typical VAD is implanted in the upper abdominal wall or attached directly to the heart. An inflow cannula drains blood from the left atrium or ventricle into a pump (part of the VAD), which then pushes the blood into the aorta through the outflow cannula.

Pump options

VADs are available as continuous flow (axial or centrifugal flow) or pulsatile pumps. A continuous flow (CF) pump fills continuously and returns blood to the aorta at a constant rate. A pulsatile pump may work in one of two ways:

1 It may fill during systole and pump blood into the aorta during diastole.

2 It may pump regardless of the patient's cardiac cycle.

Potential complications

Despite the use of anticoagulants, the VAD may cause thrombi formation, leading to pulmonary embolism or stroke. Other complications include heart failure, bleeding, cardiac tamponade, or infection.

A closer look at VADs

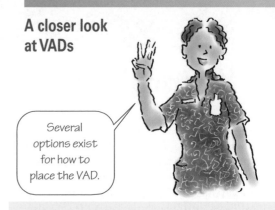

Several options exist for how to place the VAD.

Placing the VAD

VADs divert blood from failing ventricles to a pump that can effectively eject it. This diversion can occur by cannulation of either the atria or the ventricles. These illustrations show some of the cannulation options that exist.

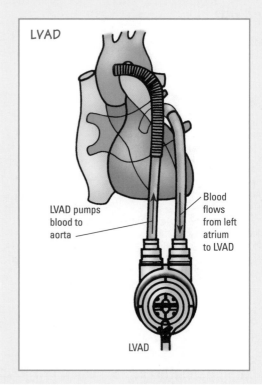

LVAD

LVAD pumps blood to aorta

Blood flows from left atrium to LVAD

LVAD

There are three types of ventricular assist device (VAD placement):

1 A right VAD (RVAD) provides pulmonary support by diverting blood from the right atrium or failing right ventricle to the VAD, which then pumps the blood to the pulmonary circulation via the VAD connection to the left pulmonary artery.

2 With a left VAD (LVAD), blood flows from the left atrium or ventricle to the VAD, which then pumps blood back to the body via the VAD connection to the aorta.

3 When an RVAD and LVAD are both used, it is referred to as *biventricular (BiVAD) support.*

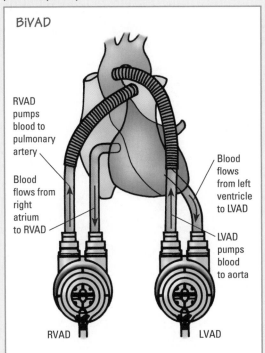

BiVAD

RVAD pumps blood to pulmonary artery

Blood flows from right atrium to RVAD

Blood flows from left ventricle to LVAD

LVAD pumps blood to aorta

RVAD   LVAD

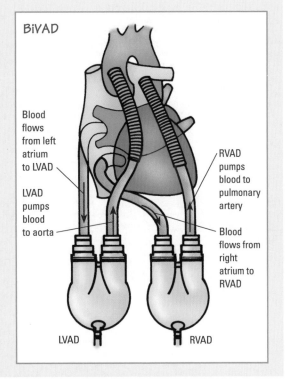

BiVAD

Blood flows from left atrium to LVAD

LVAD pumps blood to aorta

RVAD pumps blood to pulmonary artery

Blood flows from right atrium to RVAD

LVAD   RVAD

Clinical assessment

Care and assessment of patients with VADs require special attention. Equipment operation must be assessed and since patients are often discharged to home, patient education about use and care is essential. Patients will also need to be instructed about their activities of daily living such as no bathing or submersion in water (however, showering is usually allowed); care of their exit site and driveline (percutaneous lead that exits the body and connects to equipment) with scheduled sterile dressing changes and adherence to medical therapies, such as medications, labwork, and follow-up physician visits. Points about what to do in an emergency must be part of their education.

Monitoring blood pressure in continuous flow (CF) LVADs can be a challenge; normal systolic and diastolic sounds may not be heard and often the mean arterial pressure (mAP) is monitored. For example, patients with CF LVADs may need to keep their mAPs within a certain range (often less than 90 mmHg). Most VADs require patients be anticoagulated, so administration of anticoagulants and antiplatelets are critical as well as monitoring their effect (i.e., international normalized ratio or INR values). As opposed to pre-VAD implant fluid restrictions, VAD patients need to maintain adequate volume status and be well-hydrated. Lastly, monitoring for complications, such as infection, bleeding, thrombosis, and device malfunction, must be understood and communicated to health care team.

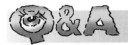

Show and tell

Identify the assessment technique being used in each illustration.

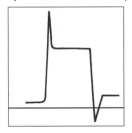 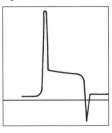 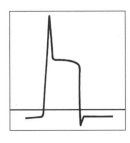 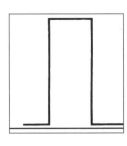

1. _____ 2. _____ 3. _____ 4. _____

True or false

VADs can be pulsatile or continuous flow

Patients with VADs can go swimming

A VAD that supports the left ventricle is called an LVAD

VADs are only used as a bridge to transplant

Question: What is monitored in VAD patients? (Check all that apply)

Blood pressure or mAP

Anticoagulation status

Signs/symptoms of infection

Understanding of VAD equipment and care

Volume or hydration status

Answers: Show and tell: 1. Balloon pressure elevation, 2. Low balloon pressure plateau, 3. Balloon pressure baseline depression, 4. High balloon pressure plateau. True or false: TRUE, FALSE, TRUE, FALSE. Question: All choices are correct.

Suggested References

Carlson, K.K. (Ed.). *AACN Advanced Critical Care Nursing.* Philadelphia: Elsevier, 2009.

Lippincott's Nursing Procedures & Skills. Philadelphia: Lippincott Williams & Wilkins, 2009. Accessed via the online program on September 1, 2009.

McLaughlin, M.A. (Ed.). *Cardiovascular Care Made Incredibly Easy,* 3rd ed. Philadelphia: Lippincott Williams & Wilkins, 2014.

Morton, P.G., and Fontaine, D.K. *Critical Care Nursing: A Holistic Approach,* 9th ed. Philadelphia: Lippincott Williams & Wilkins, 2009.

Richards, N.M., and Stahl, M.A. "Ventricular Assist Devices in the Adult," *Critical Care Nursing Quarterly* 30(2):104–118, April/June 2007.

Stahl, M., and Richards, N. "Update on Ventricular Assist Device Technology," *AACN Advanced Critical Care* 20(1):26–34, January-March 2009.

Weigand, D.L., and Carlson, K.K. *AACN Procedure Manual for Critical Care*, 6th ed. St. Louis: Elsevier Saunders, 2010.

Woods, S., et al. *Cardiac Nursing*, 6th ed. Philadelphia: Lippincott Williams & Wilkins, 2010.

Index